Chlamydial Infection: A Clinical and Public Health Perspective

Issues in Infectious Diseases

Vol. 7

Series Editor

Brian W.J. Mahy Bury St. Edmunds

Chlamydial Infection: A Clinical and Public Health Perspective

Volume Editor

Carolyn M. Black Atlanta, Ga.

12 figures, 3 in color and 12 tables, 2013

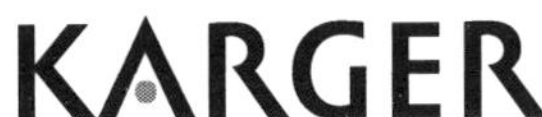

Basel · Freiburg · Paris · London · New York · New Delhi · Bangkok · Beijing · Tokyo · Kuala Lumpur · Singapore · Sydney

Issues in Infectious Diseases

Carolyn M. Black
Division of Scientific Resources
National Center for Emerging and Zoonotic
Infectious Diseases
Centers for Disease Control and Prevention
1600 Clifton Road NE
Atlanta, GA 30333(USA)

Library of Congress Cataloging-in-Publication Data

Black, Carolyn Morris.
  Chlamydial infection: a clinical and public health perspective / volume
editor, Carolyn M. Black.
      p. ; cm. -- (Issues in infectious diseases, ISSN 1660-1890 ; v. 7)
  Includes bibliographical references and indexes.
  ISBN 978-3-318-02398-5 (hard cover : alk. paper) -- ISBN 978-3-318-02399-2
(e-ISBN)
  I. Title. II. Series: Issues in infectious diseases ; v. 7. 1660-1890
  [DNLM: 1. Chlamydia Infections--physiopathology. 2. Chlamydia
trachomatis--pathogenicity. WC 600]
  RC124.5
  616.9'235--dc23

                                                                2013014316

Bibliographic Indices. This publication is listed in bibliographic services, including Current Contents® and Index Medicus.

© Copyright 2013 by S. Karger AG, P.O. Box, CH–4009 Basel (Switzerland)
© Copyright of Introduction and Chapter 7 by Carolyn M. Black, Atlanta, Ga.
www.karger.com
Printed in Germany on acid-free and non-aging paper (ISO 9706) by Stückle Druck und Verlag, Ettenheim
ISSN 1660–1890
e-ISSN 1662–3819
ISBN 978–3–318–02398–5
e-ISBN 978–3–318–02399–2

Contents

Black CM (ed): Chlamydial Infection: A Clinical and Public Health Perspective.
Issues Infect Dis. Basel, Karger, 2013, vol 7, pp 1–8 (DOI: 10.1159/000348748)

Introduction

Carolyn M. Black

Division of Scientific Resources, National Center for Emerging and Zoonotic Infectious Diseases,
Centers for Disease Control and Prevention, Atlanta, Ga., USA

Despite our knowing of it for centuries, chlamydial infection remains one of the most common bacterial infectious diseases in the world and its agent, *Chlamydia trachomatis*, is one of the most enigmatic pathogens known to medical science. This book was written to fill a dearth of books that are aimed at medical scientists and clinical practitioners who wish to delve more deeply into the clinical and public health aspects of chlamydial infection. The authors, all of whom are internationally recognized experts in this field, have provided information that is based on the latest research available at the time, in many cases including a summary of results of their own work. The book is structured in a logical fashion that begins with a description of the public health burden and epidemiology of chlamydial infections, moves through an overview of the biology and genomics of chlamydiae as they relate to the clinical spectrum and pathogenesis of infection, then reviews the topics of the immunological response, diagnosis and treatment, and finally addresses prevention with the status of current vaccine development research. We have also included a few sections on rarely presented information covering topics and populations of special interest to clinical and public health practitioners: pregnant mothers and their babies, outbreaks of a less common, invasive and systemic type of chlamydial infection known as lymphogranuloma venereum, or LGV, and chlamydial infections in men who have sex with men, gay and lesbian populations. The aim of this book is to cover clinical and public health aspects of sexually transmitted genital infections caused by *C. trachomatis* in humans and we have not attempted to cover infections caused by any other chlamydial species nor chlamydial diseases of the eye (trachoma) or respiratory tract, which have been richly described elsewhere in the literature.

To provide a backdrop for the main content of the book and for those who may be less indoctrinated in the field, the following is a short introduction on the history, biology and clinical spectrum of infections caused by *C. trachomatis*. Also, as a reference aid, it may be helpful to make note of some of the terminology used in the field to refer to this organism and its infection. The genus and species name is *Chlamydia trachomatis* (italicized), but commonly the organism is referred to as 'chlamydia' in singular and 'chlamydiae' in plural, and 'chlamydial' as an adjective, for example, 'chlamydial infection'. Use of the term 'chlamydia' or 'chlamydiae' should refer to the bacterium only; when referring to the infection caused by this bacterium, 'chlamydial infection' or 'chlamydial disease' is the more appropriate terminology.

A Short History of C. *trachomatis*

Those with interest in chlamydiae and its diseases will find that learning about the history of what has been discovered and theorized in the past provides an intriguing foreshadow of the complexity of the organism's biology and ensuing disease. A search of the literature reveals that chlamydiae were 'discovered' in 1907 but chlamydial disease had actually been known of for centuries before this. References to chlamydial-like diseases of the eye appear in ancient Egyptian and Chinese texts as early as 15 BC [1]. In 1907, the German dermatologist and radiologist Ludwig Halberstädter (1876–1949), who was reportedly one of a small number of Jewish dermatologists able to leave Nazi Germany after 1933, joined a research expedition to Java to study syphilis. It was on this expedition, in the city of Jakarta, that he joined the Austrian bacteriologist Stanislaus von Prowazek (1875–1915; fig. 1) in conducting experiments that led to the discovery of chlamydial cytoplasmic inclusion bodies in the conjunctiva of the infected eye [3]. They named these newly found inclusions 'Halberstädter-Prowazek bodies' [4], a term which has perished from use, to the relief of many. A fascinating and enigmatic photograph taken of Halberstädter and Prowazek working with a blind man holding a baby orangutan makes us wonder whether the subject of experimentation was the man or the orangutan (fig. 2).

Chlamydiae were named for the word chlamys, the ancient Greek term for the short cloak worn by Greek military men draped around their upper shoulders and secured with a brooch on the right shoulder (fig. 3). It is believed that the chlamydiae were named thus because the intracytoplasmic inclusions formed by this agent inside host cells cluster around (are 'draped' around) the nucleus of the cell (fig. 4).

Because chlamydial disease was first discovered in the eye and has a broad range of symptoms (or lack of symptoms) that resemble other diseases or syndromes, the infection was not recognized as a sexually transmitted disease until 1976 [8]. Since *C. trachomatis* is an obligate intracellular parasite (i.e. grows only inside a host cell, cannot synthesize its own ATP or grow on any artificial medium), it was believed for a long period of time to be a virus. In fact, before it was considered a virus, the cytoplasmic inclusions of *C. trachomatis* were actually mistaken for a time to be a protozoan parasite. This was perhaps the first of a long series of false starts and misunderstandings about the nature and biology of this organism that have contributed

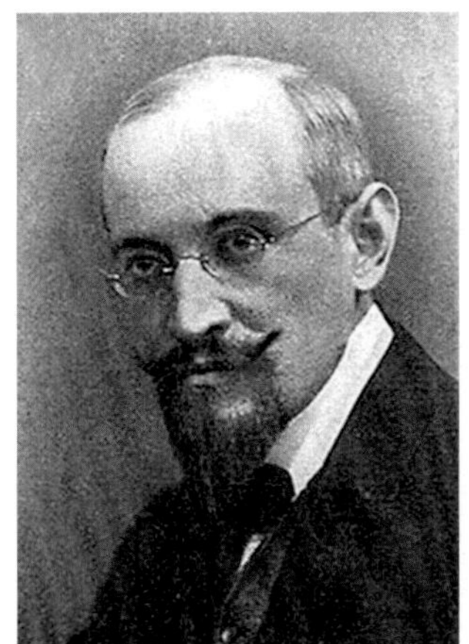

Fig. 1. Photo of Austrian bacteriologist Stanislaus von Prowazek, codiscoverer of chlamydial inclusion bodies and the cause of trachoma [2].

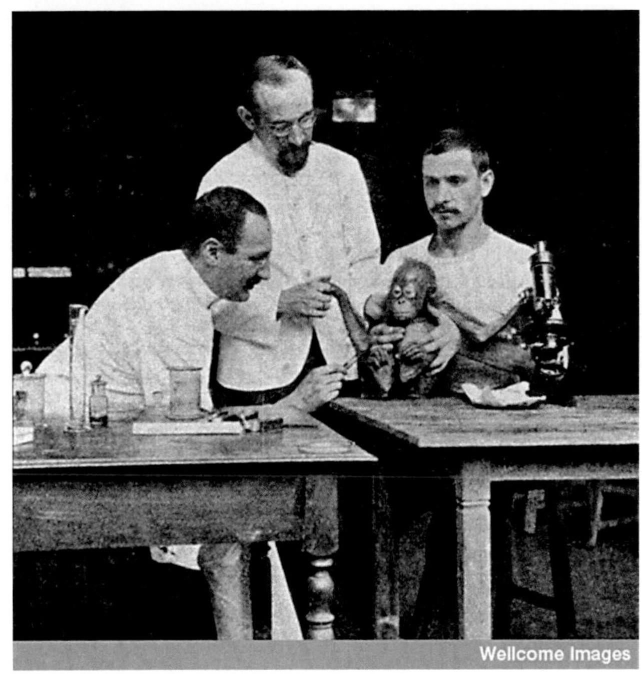

Fig. 2. Photo of Ludwig Halberstädter and Stanislaus von Prowazek (center) conducting an experiment during their research into cytoplasmic inclusion bodies of trachoma [5].

to the complexity and slow progress of research and, accordingly, the continued very high public health burden of disease [9]. Growth of the organism in embryonated eggs was first achieved in 1957 and in cell culture in 1963 – these achievements helped to finally resolve the question of whether chlamydiae were viruses or bacteria. Because of the unique developmental cycle of chlamydiae, which includes two highly distinct forms (fig. 5), the organism was classified taxonomically in a separate order (Chlamydiales).

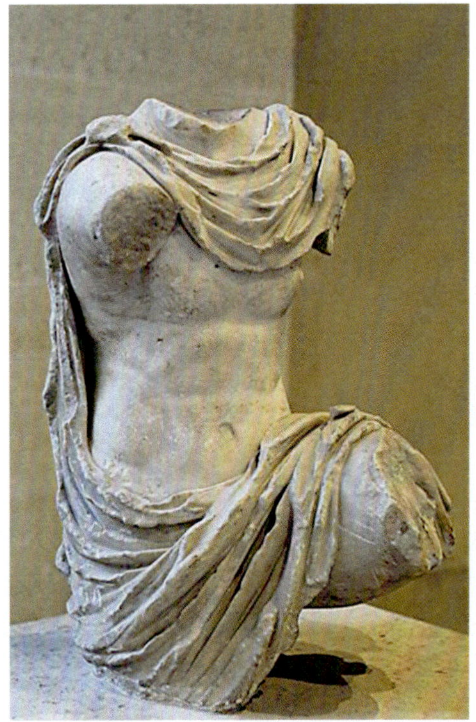

Fig. 3. Statue of a chlamys-clad figure in the Louvre Museum in Paris [6].

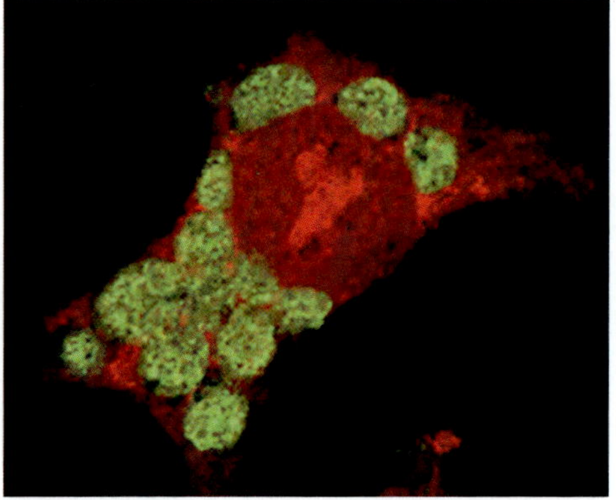

Fig. 4. Photomicrograph of fluorescently stained chlamydial inclusions (green) clustered around the nucleus of a host cell [7].

Biology and Clinical Syndromes of *C. trachomatis*

The broad clinical spectrum of infections and sequelae caused by sexually transmitted *C. trachomatis* is summarized in table 1. The infection disproportionately impacts women and the highest prevalence of infection is found in adolescent female populations. The increased susceptibility of adolescent females to *C. trachomatis* is a result of their cervical developmental stage in which the columnar epithelium protrudes through the cervical os (cervical ectopy) [15], and also due to behavioral risk factors. There are a large number of factors that contribute to the pathogenesis of chlamydiae and this topic is expertly reviewed by Deborah Dean in her chapter in this book. Since the genome of *C. trachomatis* was first sequenced and advanced sequencing technologies have subsequently permitted completion of sequencing of many strain types, significant knowledge has accumulated on the genomic structure and the contribution of chlamydial genes to the nature of infection and disease, an overview of which is included in the chapter by Tim Putman and Dan Rockey.

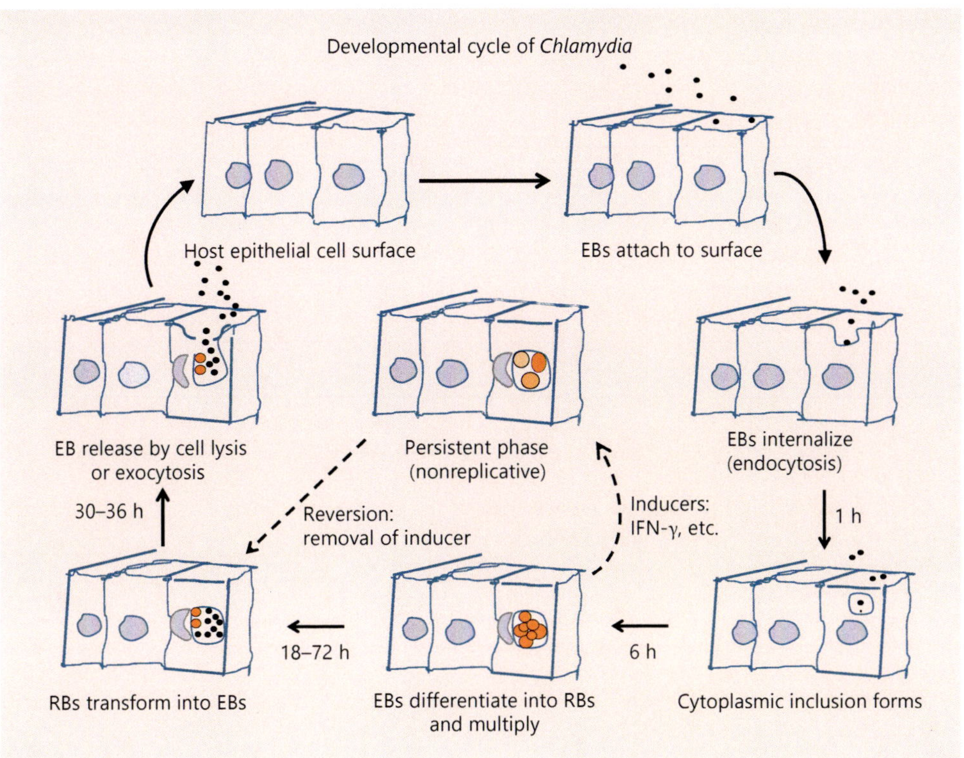

Fig. 5. Developmental cycle of chlamydiae. The infectious stage, called the elementary body (EB), infects the host epithelial cell. The EB has been loosely compared to a spore since it serves to spread or disperse itself, is metabolically inactive and has a cell wall that allows it to persist in the environment. The EB enters the host cell by endocytosis and prevents fusion of lysosomes with the chlamydia-containing phagosome, thus permitting intracellular survival. Once the phagolysosome formation is stopped, the EB secretes glycogen which induces its transition into the vegetative and noninfectious form, called the reticulate body (RB). RBs divide approximately every 2–3 h by binary fission for 18–72 h, at which point they begin to fill the endosome and are detectable by antibody-specific stain in the host cell as inclusion bodies containing 100–1,000 RBs. After division and incubation in the cytoplasmic inclusion, the RB differentiates into new infectious EBs which are released either by rupture of the host cell or by exocytosis. The RB obtains energy through straw-like structures that extend through the membrane of the inclusion into the host cell cytoplasm. There is evidence that, under certain conditions, including a host inflammatory response that produces gamma interferon (IFN-γ), the intracellular development of chlamydiae may enter an alternate path in which it becomes nonreplicative while remaining viable, this is called the persistent phase [10, 11]. For example, IFN-γ induces the depletion of tryptophan that is required for chlamydial growth leading to the 'arrest' of the developmental cycle; however, the persistent phase chlamydiae can redifferentiate into the infectious EB form and reinitiate the cycle when IFN-γ is removed or when intracellular tryptophan levels are restored. Chronic states of chlamydial disease such as trachoma and reactive arthritis may be associated with the persistent phase of the developmental cycle [12, 13].

Table 1. The clinical spectrum of sexually transmitted *C. trachomatis* infections [information from reference 14]

Females		Infants[1]	Males
lower genital tract	upper genital tract		
Asymptomatic (up to 70%)	Pelvic pain, menstrual abnormalities	Conjunctivitis	Asymptomatic (up to 50%)
Cervicitis	Pelvic inflammatory disease	Pneumonia	Nongonococcal urethritis
Urethritis	Endometritis		Epididymitis
	Salpingitis		Lymphogranuloma venereum[2]
	Pelvic peritonitis		Reiter's syndrome
	Lymphogranuloma venereum[2]		Chronic conjunctivitis
Ocular	**Sequelae**	**Sequelae**	**In men who have sex with men**
Chronic conjunctivitis	Infertility	Abnormal pulmonary function	Proctitis
	Chronic pelvic pain		Proctocolitis
	Ectopic pregnancy		
	Perihepatitis (Fitz-Hugh-Curtis syndrome)		
	Reiter's syndrome (reactive arthritis)		

[1] Refers to infants born to infected mothers.
[2] Lymphogranuloma venereum (LGV) is a chronic infection of the lymphatic system that if untreated can result in complications involving the genital organs, joints, heart, liver, eyes or, rarely, the brain. LGV is sexually transmitted but caused by different strain types of *C. trachomatis* than genital infections.

The natural history of chlamydial infection is not well understood, but it is known that up to about 70% of genital infections in women and up to 50% in men are asymptomatic. The current belief is that while some genital infections resolve without treatment, some infections persist for months to a year or more, and some may progress to serious complications such as pelvic inflammatory disease, tubal pregnancy or chronic pelvic pain. The role of host factors in the course of infection and the outcome is not very well understood and this is an exciting area of research reviewed in the chapter by Dean.

We know that chlamydial infection begins at the cervix and the urethra where it can cause cervicitis and urethritis. From the cervix, the infection may move upward into the fallopian tubes and upper genital tract, possibly by the movement of infected host macrophages bearing chlamydial inclusion bodies. It is estimated that 10–20% of untreated cervical infections lead to pelvic inflammatory disease. The presence of infection in the fallopian tubes creates a significant inflammatory response that can result in serious scarring and adhesions that affect the patency of the fallopian tube, which leads to infertility. Chlamydial infections are highly prevalent in adolescent populations, who commonly become infected more than once, especially when their sexual partners are not treated. The epidemiology and control of chlamydial infections is described in detail in this book in the chapter by Catherine Satterwhite and John Douglas. The host response to infection is now understood as playing a critical role in the pathogenesis of infection – this phenomenon and a detailed review of the immunology of chlamydial infection is included here in a chapter by Ray Johnson and Will Geisler.

Although there are sophisticated diagnostic tests available for chlamydial infections (described in detail in the chapter by Charlotte Gaydos), a large number of infected people do not present for medical care since they have no symptoms and are unaware of being infected. They are thus important sources of spread of infection to others. Laboratory testing followed by treatment is currently the best approach for the control of chlamydial infections. Investigations that seek to identify a virulence factor or factors that might prove to be effective vaccine candidates have been conducted for about 2 decades but have proved elusive to date (reviewed here by Joseph Igietseme and Carolyn Black). Antimicrobial treatment regimens for chlamydial infection and its complications are generally considered to be effective and are described in the chapter in this book by Margaret Hammerschlag.

No treatise on the public health aspects of chlamydial infection would be complete without attention to some of the populations who are disproportionately or uniquely affected by this sexually transmitted disease. Toward this end, Ingrid Rours and Margaret Hammerschlag have contributed a chapter on complications of chlamydial infections in babies born to infected mothers, Henry de Vries and Servaas Morré have described an intriguing cluster of infections in men who have sex with men, and Devika Singh and Jeanne Marazzo have contributed a chapter on chlamydial infections in gay and lesbian populations.

Acknowledgments

I am grateful to the authors for their willingness to spend their valuable time and effort in making exceptional contributions to this work. Their passion for the often arduous and intricate work involved in the study of this pathogen is evident in their writing. I am also grateful to Dr. Claudiu Bandea for his insightful review, critique and suggestions for improvement. It is my hope that this book will not only inform and assist clinicians and public health providers, but also peak the curiosity of and inspire rich endeavors by the chlamydiologists of the future.

Disclaimer

References

1 Taylor HR: Trachoma: A Blinding Scourge from the Bronze Age to the Twenty-First Century. Melbourne, Centre for Eye Research Australia, 2008.
2 Photo from Wikimedia Commons, a freely licensed media repository. http://en.wikipedia.org/wiki/File: Prowazek.jpg
3 Von Prowazek S, Halberstädter L: Zur Aetiologie des Trachoms. Dtsch Med Wochenschr 1907;33:1285–1287.
4 Whonamedit?: A Dictionary for Medical Eponyms: Halberstädter-Prowazek bodies. http://www.whonamedit.com/synd.cfm/3980.html.
5 Photo from Welcome Trust Illustrated history of tropical diseases. Wellcome Images Ref No. GC LA/Ill, http://images.wellcome.ac.uk. Wellcome Library, London.
6 Photo from Wikimedia Commons, a freely licensed media repository. http://en.wikipedia.org/wiki/File: Chlamys-clad_figure_Louvre_Ma305_n2.jpg.
7 Photo reproduced with permission from Prof. Dr. Thomas Miethke, Institut für Medizinische, Mikrobiologie, Immunologie und Hygiene, Munich, Germany.
8 Schachter J, Causse G, Tarizzo ML: Chlamydiae as agents of sexually transmitted disease. WHO Bulletin 1976;54:245–254.
9 World Health Organisation: World Health Report, 2001. Geneva, WHO, 2001.
10 Beatty WL, Morrison RP, Byrne GI: Persistent chlamydiae: from cell culture to a paradigm for chlamydial pathogenesis. Microbiol Rev 1994;58:686–699.
11 Morrison RP: New insights into a persistent problem – chlamydial infections. J Clin Invest 2003;111: 1647–1649.
12 Beatty WL, Byrne GI, Morrison RP: Repeated and persistent infection with *Chlamydia* and the development of chronic inflammation and disease. Trends Microbiol 1994;2:94–98.
13 Villareal C, Whittum-Hudson JA, Hudson AP: Persistent Chlamydiae and chronic arthritis. Arthritis Res 2002;4:5–9.
14 Centers for Disease Control and Prevention: Recommendations for the prevention and management of *Chlamydia trachomatis* infections, 1993. Atlanta, MMWR, 1993.
15 Lee V, Tobin JM, Foley E: Relationship of cervical ectopy to chlamydial infection in young women. J Fam Plann Reprod Health Care 2006;32:104–106.

Dr. Carolyn M. Black
Division of Scientific Resources, National Center for Emerging and Zoonotic Infectious Diseases
Centers for Disease Control and Prevention
Atlanta, GA 30333 (USA)
E-Mail cblack@cdc.gov

Chapter 1

Black CM (ed): Chlamydial Infection: A Clinical and Public Health Perspective.
Issues Infect Dis. Basel, Karger, 2013, vol 7, pp 9–24 (DOI: 10.1159/000348750)

Epidemiology and Prevention and Control Programs for Chlamydia

Catherine L. Satterwhite · John M. Douglas, Jr.

Division of STD Prevention and National Center for HIV, Viral Hepatitis, STD, and TB Prevention,
Centers for Disease Control and Prevention, Atlanta, Ga., USA

Abstract

An estimated 2.9 million cases of *Chlamydia trachomatis* occur annually in the USA, and while most infections are not detected and reported, chlamydia is the most commonly reported nationally notifiable disease in the USA, with over 1.2 million cases reported in 2009. Rates of reported cases of chlamydia have increased over the past decade as a result of expanded use of more sensitive diagnostic tests and increased testing. The highest case rates are in adolescents/young adults, females and African-Americans. In contrast to increases in reported case rates, prevalence in routinely tested populations appears to be stable in some settings (e.g. women tested in family planning clinics) and declining in others (e.g. high-risk youths assessed by the National Job Training Program, the general population assessed by the National Health and Nutrition Examination Survey). Prevention and control programs rely on detection and treatment of infection to prevent complications and ongoing transmission, based primarily on recommended annual screening of young sexually active women and treatment of sex partners. Important complementary prevention components include enhancing awareness to promote adherence to recommended testing and education and risk reduction counseling to promote condom use. Enhancing the public health impact of chlamydia prevention and control requires expanding population coverage of recommended strategies, especially among the most affected populations.

Current Burden of Infection

An estimated 2.9 million cases of *Chlamydia trachomatis* infection occur annually in the USA [1]. However, many of these infections are not detected and treated. Despite this, chlamydia is still the most commonly reported nationally notifiable disease [2]. Chlamydia was made a nationally notifiable disease in 1995 and was reported by all states by 2000. In 2009, over 1.2 million cases were reported; four times more chlamydia cases were reported than gonorrhea cases, the next most frequently reported notifiable disease [3].

Chlamydia may lead to serious adverse outcomes among women, including pelvic inflammatory disease (PID), ectopic pregnancy, tubal-factor infertility and chronic pelvic pain. Among men, chlamydia may result in urethritis, prostatitis and epididymitis. The frequency of occurrence, asymptomatic nature of infection and the possibility of adverse outcomes prompted the development of widespread screening recommendations for women in 1993 [4]. Currently, annual chlamydia screening is recommended for all sexually active women aged 25 years or younger [5]. Rates of reported chlamydia are highest among young women, reflecting these screening recommendations. Among women aged 14–19 years, the 2009 reported chlamydia rate was 3,329.3 cases per 100,000 population; among women aged 20–24, the rate was 3,273.9. Reported case rates among men are substantially lower (in 2009, 1,120.6 cases per 100,000 men aged 20–24 years). Lower reported rates in men are likely due to lower rates of testing and detection of chlamydial infections in this population, when compared to broad screening among women. Racial disparities exist in reported chlamydia rates, likely related at least in part to social determinants of health such as poverty, access to healthcare and living in communities with high STD prevalence: in 2009, black men and women were over eight times more likely than white men and women to have a reported case of chlamydia [3].

An analysis of chlamydia data from 1999 to 2002 from the National Health and Nutrition Examination Survey (NHANES), a continuous population-based survey conducted annually, showed that overall chlamydia prevalence among the general population of US men and women aged 14–39 years was 2.0% (95% confidence interval, CI, 1.6–2.5%) [6]. NHANES consists of annual data on approximately 5,000 US, noninstitutionalized men and women, selected using complex sampling methodology. Stratified by age group, chlamydia prevalence was highest among young men and women aged 20–29 years (3.2%). As with case report data, non-Hispanic blacks bore a disproportionate burden of infection with a prevalence of 5.3%, compared to a 1.5% prevalence among white men and women. The prevalence of infection was similar among men (2.0%) and women (2.5%), contrary to case reports which are more likely to reflect screening practices. In a more recent NHANES analysis limited to sexually active adolescent women aged 14–19 years, chlamydia prevalence was 7.1% [7].

Epidemiologic Trends

While estimates of chlamydial infection provide a comprehensive picture of current burden, assessing longitudinal trends are essential when considering a possible impact of prevention efforts. However, interpreting chlamydia trends is challenging. When examining trends, two important factors must be considered: changes in test technology utilization and changes in screening coverage.

Chlamydia Test Technology

Chlamydia test technology has substantially changed over time. The current optimal test technology utilized to detect genital *C. trachomatis* infections is a nucleic acid amplification test (NAAT) [8]. No true gold standard test for chlamydia exists; however, NAAT performance is superior to the traditional gold standard, *C. trachomatis* culture [9], with estimated sensitivity of greater than 90% and specificity levels of approximately 99% [8]. First introduced in the late 1990s, NAAT technology usage was initially cost prohibitive. However, as costs were reduced and additional studies demonstrated clear advancements over prior generation tests, usage increased. In 2000, 24.5% of all chlamydia tests conducted in surveyed public health laboratories in the USA were NAATs [10]; by 2007, this proportion had increased to 81.6% [11].

While improvements in test technology have been advantageous for diagnosis, they present significant challenges in determining and interpreting epidemiologic trends. The increased sensitivity of newer tests has resulted in better detection of existing infections; older test technologies likely missed infections due to reduced sensitivity [12]. If test type is not considered, increases in chlamydia rates due to use of more sensitive tests may incorrectly appear to represent increases in actual disease burden. Studies have demonstrated the impact of test technology in estimating chlamydia prevalence. Dicker et al. [12] found that chlamydia positivity in Philadelphia family planning clinics increased by 46% when NAATs replaced DNA probes (from 4.1 to 6.0%). Likewise, an analysis of data from the National Job Training Program (NJTP) revealed a 1-year increase (2005–2006) in prevalence from 9.1 to 13.9% (53% increase) associated with a dramatic shift in test technology: from 2005 to 2006, NAAT usage went from 21 to 88% of all tests [13]. When chlamydia trends were assessed, prevalence in the NJTP increased between 2003 and 2007, but after adjustment for test technology and other confounding factors, a statistically significant decrease was reported, highlighting the importance of test technology in interpreting chlamydia surveillance trends.

Chlamydia Screening Recommendations

Screening recommendations for young sexually active women have been in place since 1993 [4]. Currently, the Centers for Disease Control and Prevention (CDC) recommends that all sexually active women under the age of 26 years be screened annually for chlamydia [5]. In addition, the US Preventive Services Task Force (USPSTF) has recommended screening of young, sexually active women since 2001 [14]. In 2007, USPSTF updated their chlamydia screening recommendations to change the upper age bound from under 26 years to under 25 years of age, a change from the CDC-recommended upper age range [15] made to be consistent with nationally reported surveillance data age groupings [16]. Both CDC and USPSTF also recommend chlamydia screening for older women with risk factors. In sum, both the CDC and USPSTF, as well as most major medical organizations, uniformly recommend

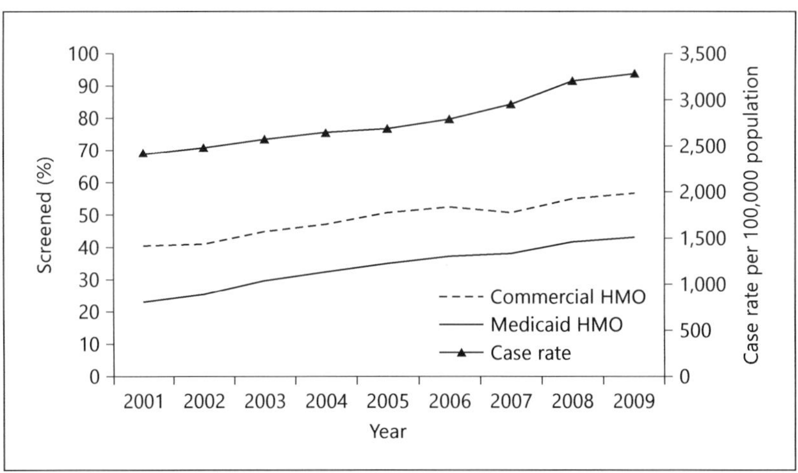

Fig. 1. Chlamydia screening coverage and chlamydia case report rates, women aged 15–24 years, 2001–2009. Sources: US national chlamydia morbidity data [C. Satterwhite, pers. commun.] and The State of Healthcare Quality, 2010 [19]. In 2001, screening coverage data are for women aged 16–26 years; from 2002–2007, women aged 16–25 years and from 2008–2009, women aged 16–24 years. Screening coverage is among women seeking healthcare who are considered to be sexually active. HMO = Health maintenance organization.

that young, sexually active women under the age of 25 years be screened annually for chlamydia [17].

The National Committee for Quality Assurance added chlamydia screening coverage among women as a measure in the Healthcare Effectiveness Data and Information Set (HEDIS) in 1999 [18]. Chlamydia screening coverage, as measured by HEDIS, has increased steadily over time. Between 2001 and 2009, screening coverage among young women (aged 16–26 years in 2001; 16–25 years from 2002 to 2007; 16–24 years from 2008 to 2009) who were enrolled in a commercial healthcare plan and had a visit where they were determined to be sexually active increased substantially, from 23.1 to 43.1% (fig. 1) [19]. Overall, coverage was consistently higher among Medicaid populations when compared to commercial populations, and from 2001 to 2009 coverage in the Medicaid population increased from 40.4 to 56.7%. Increasing chlamydia screening coverage has undoubtedly had a substantial impact on trends in reported cases, since, as more women are screened, more existing cases are detected (fig. 1).

Epidemiologic Trends in Chlamydial Infection

For the past 20 years, reported overall chlamydia case rates (all ages, both sexes) have steadily increased in the USA, from 160.2 cases per 100,000 population in 1990 to 409.2 cases per 100,000 in 2009 [3]. With continued increases in screening, data system enhancements and use of increasingly sensitive tests, ongoing increases in the

Satterwhite · Douglas

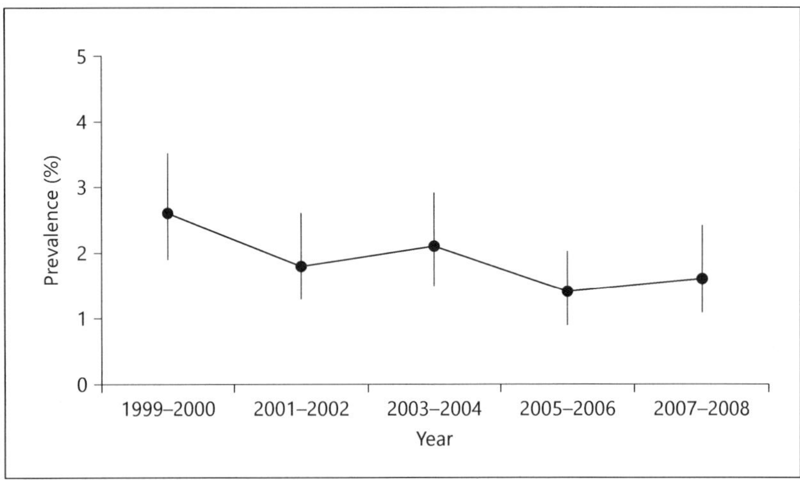

Fig. 2. Chlamydia prevalence among men and women aged 14–39 years, NHANES, USA, 1999–2008. Bars indicate 95% CI. Produced from data published in Datta et al. [21].

number of chlamydia cases reported are expected. Since case report data do not necessarily represent trends in disease burden, but rather trends in case detection, population-based prevalence data in defined populations undergoing consistent testing are more useful in assessing epidemiologic trends [20].

When results from NHANES, in a sample considered to be representative of the general population, were examined over time, chlamydia prevalence significantly decreased between 1999 and 2008, from 2.6% (95% CI: 1.9, 3.5) in 1999/2000 to 1.6% in 2007/2008 (95% CI: 1.1, 2.4; fig. 2) [21]. Of note, while NHANES is an important source of chlamydia prevalence trend data, the stability of point estimates will fall if prevalence continues to decrease and standard errors increase, thus limiting this survey's ability to detect changes in prevalence over time.

Prevalence trends can also be monitored in clinic-based surveys. The Infertility Prevention Project (IPP) is a national program administered primarily through family planning clinics, targeting young women for chlamydia screening. Test-based data reported through IPP are used to calculate chlamydia positivity (positive tests/total tests), with positivity shown to closely approximate prevalence [22]. State IPP positivity varies substantially and is highest in the southeast, consistent with case rates [3]. Among women attending family planning clinics aged 15–24 years, median state-specific IPP chlamydia positivity has steadily increased over time, between 1997 and 2009 [3]. However, similar to morbidity data, NAAT usage has increased in IPP, so crude positivity has been impacted by improvements in test technology. In a recent multivariate analysis of IPP data, trends were assessed using a clinic-based analysis taking test technology and other population characteristics into account [23]. This analysis showed that positivity remained unchanged in family planning clinics from

2004 to 2008. In contrast, among women aged 15–24 years tested in prenatal clinics, where testing is routinely recommended and thus the population tested is less likely to be influenced by perceived STD risk, positivity declined from 2004 to 2009, similar to NHANES findings [24].

Finally, data from the NJTP, a program serving young, socio-economically disadvantaged men and women aged 16–24 years, are not subject to some of the limitations present in case report and IPP data. Nearly all NJTP participants are screened for chlamydia at program entrance, using consistent test technology [13]; thus, the population is defined and routinely tested in a standardized way. Chlamydia prevalence is high; in 2009, the median state-specific prevalence was 11.3% among women and 7.0% among men [3]. While NJTP data represent a high-risk population not broadly generalizable, this relatively consistent population (stable demographics and social characteristics) provides important insight into the national chlamydia burden. Consistent with NHANES and IPP prenatal clinic data, significant decreases in chlamydia prevalence have been detected in the young at-risk men and women entering the NJTP over three consecutive time periods: from 1990 to 1997 [25], from 1998 to 2004 [26] and, most recently, from 2003 to 2007 [13].

Importance and Challenges of Monitoring Sequelae of Infection

PID is the most immediate important adverse outcome of chlamydial infection in women. Untreated chlamydia leads to PID in approximately 10–15% of cases [27, 28]. In turn, PID may lead to further sequelae, including tubal-factor infertility, ectopic pregnancy and chronic pelvic pain [29], although the specific contribution of chlamydia to each is unknown [30] since chlamydia is only one of many possible causes. However, given that the primary objective of prevention programs is to reduce these sequelae, monitoring their trends is an important consideration in understanding the impact of chlamydia prevention and control efforts.

In the absence of a laboratory-based case definition, the diagnosis of PID is based upon clinical signs and symptoms [5]. This diagnosis lacks specificity and is not easily standardized; thus, trends in PID diagnoses are difficult to interpret. At the national level, data for monitoring PID trends are routinely obtained from complex sample surveys, as well as surveys of administrative data, including hospital admissions. While each of these data sources has limitations, all suggest a downward trend in PID diagnoses [3]. Similarly, a recent analysis of administrative data from a national insurance claims database also revealed decreases [31].

Challenges also exist when considering trends in ectopic pregnancy and infertility. Ectopic pregnancy is more easily diagnosed than PID, but more distal from a possibly causal chlamydia infection, complicating interpretation of prevention effort impact. In addition, ectopic pregnancy is increasingly managed in the outpatient setting [32], making the consistent declines seen in hospitalizations over the past decade difficult to interpret [3]. A recent analysis of administrative claims data, taking into account both inpatient and outpatient data, showed stable ectopic pregnancy rates in the USA from 2002 to 2007 [32]. Infertility, like ectopic pregnancy, is a relatively distal outcome following chlamydia and is even more difficult to monitor since, in order to be diagnosed, healthcare must be sought, which implies both the desire to have a baby and access to services, including ability to incur costs. Nonetheless, an analysis of data from the National Survey of Family Growth, 1982–2002, showed a decline in 12-month self-reported infertility among women [33].

International Chlamydia Trends

As noted, in the USA, a variety of data sources show that chlamydia prevalence is stable or decreasing, not increasing as might be suggested by national case report trends. In Sweden and British Columbia, Canada, where chlamydia screening programs also exist, similar increases in case report trends have been reported [34–36] and have been hypothesized to be related either to screening of insufficient magnitude to effectively reduce disease incidence or, alternatively, reduced population immunity as a paradoxical result of successful screening, leading to increased susceptibility to reinfection, a phenomenon termed 'arrested immunity' [35–37]. Analyses using alternate data sources, such as the prevalence surveys available in the USA, have not been conducted, so the impact of factors such as test technology changes and increasing screening coverage have not been well studied.

Chlamydia Prevention and Control

The rationale for public health programs to prevent and control chlamydial infection is the high burden of infection, and the role of chlamydia as a major preventable cause of costly reproductive morbidity in women. Prevention efforts for chlamydia depend on both primary prevention (preventing infection and ongoing transmission) and secondary prevention (preventing complications in those infected). The transmission of STDs within a population depends upon several factors, summarized by the formula $R_0 = BcD$, where the reproductive rate (R_0, the average number of new infections that an infected individual generates) is a function of the average probability of transmission from an infected to a susceptible partner (B), the average number of sexual partnerships formed over time between infected and susceptible partners (c) and the duration of infectiousness (D). Incidence and prevalence increase within a population when R_0 exceeds 1, and they decrease when it falls below 1. Primary prevention approaches are based on decreasing one or more of these transmission parameters, such as reducing the efficiency of transmission (i.e. using condoms), reducing the number of partners, or, most importantly, reducing the duration of infection by treating index patients and their sexual partners. Treatment with effective antimicrobial therapy, prompted by positive diagnostic or screening tests or given empirically to those with a high likelihood of infection, is also the mainstay of secondary prevention.

Case Detection and Treatment

As outlined later in this book, chlamydia infections can be easily diagnosed and treated. Urogenital infections in women can be detected by testing samples such as urine or swabs from the cervix or vagina, while those in men can be detected by testing urine or urethral swabs; rectal and pharyngeal infections can be detected using swabs from these sites. At all anatomic sites, testing by NAAT is preferred over other tests due to greater sensitivity [8]. Recommended treatment includes single doses of azithromycin or 1-week courses of doxycycline, which are estimated to have microbial cure rates of 97 and 98%, respectively [5]. Diagnostic testing for suspected infection, with empiric therapy pending test results, is indicated for a variety of chlamydia-associated clinical syndromes (e.g. cervicitis, urethritis, epididymitis, PID and proctitis) and for sexual partners of persons with suspected or proven infection [5]. Promptly administered treatment can reduce the likelihood of PID in women with cervicitis and of longer-term sequelae in those with PID [5, 38].

Screening for Prevention

Because most chlamydial infections are asymptomatic, screening tests performed in the absence of clinical findings is the most important approach to detection of infection and is a key strategy for prevention and control programs. As noted above, annual testing of sexually active young women (<25 years old) and older women with risk factors is recommended by the CDC and USPSTF [5, 15], and ranked by the National Commission on Prevention Priorities as one of the highest priorities of all clinical preventive services, based on cost effectiveness and clinically preventable burden, and also one of the most underutilized [39]. A number of other countries have implemented chlamydia screening programs among young women including Canada, the UK, the Netherlands and several Scandinavian countries [34, 40].

Screening recommendations are primarily based on the benefit of screening for secondary prevention, by enhancing early detection and treatment of chlamydia infection and preventing complications, such as PID [14]. This rationale is similar to that for other prevention strategies such as cervical cancer screening via Pap testing, where long-term complications of an infectious disease (i.e. human papillomavirus infection) are prevented through a secondary prevention approach. Several randomized clinical trials have shown reductions in PID among young women undergoing chlamydia screening, including women in a US health maintenance organization (estimated reduction of 56%) [41] and Dutch high school students undergoing home-based testing (estimated reduction 50%) [42]. In addition, a recent trial of chlamydia screening among college/university students in the UK found an estimated reduction in PID of 35%, although the difference was not statistically significant [28]. Using a different design, a nonrandomized ecologic study found lower rates of PID (estimated reduction of 39%) in American military servicewoman who were screened at the time of recruit training (in the US Navy) compared to those who were not (in the US Army) [43]. These studies primarily assessed cases of PID occurring in the outpatient setting; in contrast, given the often mild nature of chlamydial PID, a study comparing rates of hospitalization for PID among US Army women found no difference among those who were screened for chlamydia versus those who were not [44]. In addition, consistent with findings from clinical trials, several surveillance analyses have reported declines in PID and other sequelae following the introduction of chlamydia screening [31, 37, 45–49]. However, as noted above, attributing trends in complications such as PID at the population level to the impact of screening programs is challenging given diagnostic imprecision and the fact that not all PID is caused by chlamydia.

In spite of this apparent secondary prevention benefit, questions about the value of chlamydia screening programs have been raised because reductions in incidence and prevalence following their introduction have not been consistently seen, as would be expected if they also had primary prevention benefit in reducing ongoing transmission and as had been seen decades earlier with gonorrhea control programs [20, 34–36, 50, 51]. As noted above, possible explanations for the lack of declining rates after initiation of screening include increased testing and increased use of more sensitive diagnostic tests resulting in greater numbers of reported cases, insufficient screening coverage of the population, or arrested immunity [20, 34, 36, 37]. These findings have led to calls for randomized trials of screening programs to assess the impact on population chlamydia prevalence, as a more precise outcome than PID, and trials to address this question, in settings where current lack of recommendations for widespread screening make it ethically feasible to study, are now underway [52].

Improving Population Outcomes and Screening Coverage
While estimated coverage of recommended screening by eligible females has been increasing (fig. 1), it remains suboptimal. It is likely that coverage assessments as measured in HEDIS are overestimates [18] because of underestimation in the administrative data on which the estimates are based of women for whom testing is indicated (i.e. sexually active women). In addition, because HEDIS measures assess screening only in insured women who have accessed care, it is only representative of this group, which does not include women not seeking care or who lack insurance; lack of insurance is known to be associated with reduced levels of screening [53]. A

recent analysis of claims data indicates that with a more representative estimation of eligible women, screening rates may be as low as half the level estimated by HEDIS [54]. Improving screening coverage will involve addressing barriers at the level of both the provider and the patient. Provider issues include reluctance to routinely assess sexual history among adolescents, perception that patients in their setting are at low risk of chlamydia and unfamiliarity with testing of specimens not requiring a pelvic examination (e.g. vaginal swabs and urine samples). In addition to lack of insurance, patient issues include lack of knowledge of the recommendation for annual chlamydia testing and limited understanding of the asymptomatic nature and potential long-term complications of chlamydia infection [18, 55]. In the USA, the recently formed National Chlamydia Coalition is addressing barriers to chlamydia screening at the provider, patient and policy level (http://ncc.prevent.org). A particularly promising example of a social marketing campaign to increase testing for STDs including chlamydia is the 'GYT' (Get Yourself Talking/Get Yourself Tested) campaign (http://www.gytnow.org) that aims to normalize communication and use of preventive services for sexual health, and has been associated with substantial increases in testing at sentinel clinics across the USA [56]. Finally, the recently passed Affordable Care Act in the USA has the potential to increase testing both because of increased numbers of individuals who may be covered by insurance as well as mandatory provision of preventive services recommended by the USPSTF without required copayment by patients.

Screening among Males
Although chlamydia testing is recommended for diagnosis among men with suspected infection based on clinical findings or exposure to an infected partner, CDC and USPSTF do not recommend routine screening of sexually active young men in the general population because of insufficient evidence of its impact in decreasing incidence in women and cost effectiveness [15]. However, CDC advises consideration of male screening in clinical settings with a high chlamydia prevalence, such as adolescent and STD clinics and correctional facilities, where screening will be more cost effective [5, 57]. In addition, among men who have sex with men, because of high prevalence and the potential for reducing HIV transmission, CDC recommends annual screening for STDs, including chlamydia, based on history of recent sexual activity (i.e. urine testing if insertive sex and rectal testing if receptive anal sex), with more frequent testing in those with greater risk (multiple or anonymous partners, illicit drug use) [5].

Rescreening after Treatment
Increasing data indicate a high prevalence of recurrent infection in both women and men following treatment for chlamydia, with estimates ranging from 13 to 18% [58, 59]. Because recurrent infections increase the risk of PID in women and ongoing transmission in both women and men, it is recommended that individuals treated for

chlamydia be retested approximately 3 months after treatment or at the first clinical opportunity thereafter [5]. Although limited attempts to enhance retesting via postal reminders have not been effective, electronic reminders (email, text messages) may be more promising [60].

Special Populations
Adolescents. Chlamydia screening is particularly important in adolescents because of their high rates of infection [3, 6] and because they have the longest timeframe over which to experience long-term complications such as infertility. Special challenges in this population include the failure of providers to discuss sexual behaviors and provide recommended services such as risk reduction counseling and chlamydia screening. In addition, while adolescents may consent for their own sexual health services in all states, protecting confidentiality can be an issue for those covered by private insurance since many states mandate that health plans provide an 'explanation of benefits' to the beneficiary (typically the parent) of services covered. To address this issue, professional organizations have developed coding and billing tools to maximize reimbursement while minimizing potential disclosure of confidential services through health plan billing statements (http://www.adolescenthealth.org/Clinical_Care_Resources/2304.htm).

Pregnant Females (see the chapter by Rours and Hammerschlag). Chlamydia infection in pregnant women can result in complications in pregnancy (e.g. prematurity and postpartum endometritis) and postpartum infection in infants (e.g. conjunctivitis and pneumonia). CDC recommends screening all pregnant women during their first prenatal visit and retesting those at risk of new or recurrent infections in the third trimester (e.g. women aged <25 years, or those who have new or multiple partners or chlamydia diagnosed earlier in pregnancy) [5].

Persons with HIV Infection. Testing for chlamydia and other STDs is recommended at the initial medical evaluation of persons with HIV infection at anatomic sites of recent sexual exposure. Testing is also recommended annually for sexually active HIV-positive individuals, for both personal health benefit and also to reduce the possibility of enhanced HIV transmission due to untreated STDs. In addition, a positive test for chlamydia or other STI indicates sexual behavior that could transmit HIV and should prompt risk-reduction counseling [5].

Partner Services

As for other bacterial STDs, notifying and treating partners of persons with presumed or confirmed chlamydial infection has long been recommended as a core prevention strategy in order to prevent reinfection of the index case, morbidity in the partner and ongoing transmission. CDC recommends that partners with sexual contact within 60 days of diagnosis or onset of symptoms should be treated [5]. The importance of partner treatment is highlighted by a recent modeling study which indicated that increasing rates of partner treatment could have a greater impact on reducing population prevalence than increasing screening rates [61]. Approaches based on referral of partners by patients are likely less effective than provider referral, although the high chlamydia caseload makes the latter impractical in most jurisdictions, and it is likely that provider referral is offered to only a minority of persons with chlamydia [62].

Given this reality, there has been growing interest in alternative approaches, particularly expedited partner therapy (EPT), a process in which the index patient delivers a prescription or medication directly to their partner(s) without the need for clinical assessment of the partner [63]. Use of EPT is associated with higher rates of reported partner treatment and lower rates of reinfection in the index patient [64]. Although EPT is a promising approach, there are several barriers to its widespread use. Providing medication to a person with whom the provider has no professional relationship is not legal in some jurisdictions of the USA, although the number of states in which EPT is permissible has been increasing (http://www.cdc.gov/std/ept/legal/default.htm). In addition, there are implementation issues, such as reluctance of payers to provide medications for partners not covered by their plan. Another promising partner services strategy is encouraging persons who test positive at screening to bring in their partners at the time they return for treatment; this 'BYOP' (bring your own partner) approach results in rates of partner treatment similar to those for EPT [65]. Finally, an additional challenge for EPT and other partner services approaches is how best to monitor their provision at the population level.

Primary Prevention

In addition to detecting and treating persons with chlamydia to prevent ongoing infection, other modalities are important for primary prevention. Behavioral risk reduction interventions have been proven to reduce new infections with chlamydia and other STDs, and CDC and USPSTF recommend high-intensity behavioral counseling for all sexually active adolescents and adults at risk for STD [5, 66]. The benefit of such counseling is likely mediated by partner reduction and also increased utilization of condoms. Correct and consistent condom use can reduce the risk for chlamydia [5] and may also reduce the risk for PID; one study reported that condom use in women with prior PID reduced the incidence of recurrent PID, chronic pelvic pain and infertility [67]. In addition, female-controlled barriers such as the diaphragm and female condom may also reduce the risk of chlamydia and other STDs [68]. Finally, available data are conflicting regarding whether male circumcision will prevent chlamydia in males or their partners [69].

Conclusion

Prevention and control of chlamydia remains a major priority in the USA and other countries. While many challenges persist in optimizing the impact of prevention programs, emerging data from one of the most effective approaches for assessing program impact – sequential prevalence studies of nonclinic-based populations whose testing is not influenced by healthcare-seeking behavior [20] – are beginning to indicate declines in prevalence in the USA (fig. 2) [13, 21, 23]. While these trends could be influenced by other factors such as changes in sexual behavior [70], they are consistent with the impact of prevention programs, and they could accelerate if population coverage of screening and partner services increases [61]. As outlined in the following chapter, there are many gaps in our understanding of the natural history and immunology of *C. trachomatis* infection (e.g. the relative importance of persistent infection vs. recently acquired infection or reinfection in causing PID and long-term sequelae) which affect the optimal structure of prevention and control programs. For example, annual screening as currently recommended may have greater impact on sequelae resulting from persistent infection, while partner treatment and early retesting after treatment may be more effective in preventing or detecting recently acquired infection [71]. Until these issues can be resolved, prevention and control programs should attempt to optimize each of the prevention components outlined above to provide increasing population impact.

References

1 Satterwhite CL, Torrone E, Meites E, Dunne EF, Mahajan R, Banez Ocfemia C, Su J, Xu F, Weinstock H: Sexually transmitted infections among U.S. women and men: Prevalence and incidence estimates, 2008. Sex Transm Dis 2013;40:187–193.

2 Centers for Disease Control and Prevention: Summary of notifiable diseases – United States, 2007. MMWR Morb Mortal Wkly Rep 2007;56:22.

3 Centers for Disease Control and Prevention: Sexually Transmitted Disease Surveillance, 2009. Atlanta, US Department of Health and Human Services, 2010.

4 Centers for Disease Control and Prevention: Recommendations for the prevention and management of *Chlamydia trachomatis* infections, 1993. MMWR Recomm Rep 1993;42:1–38.

5 Workowski KA, Berman S, Centers for Disease Control and Prevention: Sexually transmitted diseases treatment guidelines, 2010. MMWR Recomm Rep 2010;59:1–110.

6 Datta SD, Sternberg M, Johnson RE, Berman S, Papp JR, McQuillan G, Weinstock H: Gonorrhea and chlamydia in the United States among persons 14 to 39 years of age, 1999 to 2002. Ann Intern Med 2007;147:89–96.

7 Forhan S, Gottlieb S, Sternberg M, Xu F, Datta SD, McQuillan G, Berman S, Markowitz L: Prevalence of sexually transmitted infections among female adolescents aged 14 to 19 in the United States. Pediatrics 2009;124:1505–1512.

8 Association of Public Health Laboratories: Laboratory diagnostic testing for *Chlamydia trachomatis* and *Neisseria gonorrhoeae*: expert consultation meeting summary report. http://www.aphl.org/aphlprograms/infectious/std/Documents/CTGCLabGuidelinesMeetingReport.pdf (accessed March, 2011).

9 Hadgu A, Dendukuri N, Hilden J: Evaluation of nucleic acid amplification tests in the absence of a perfect gold-standard test: a review of the statistical and epidemiologic issues. Epidemiology 2005;16:604–612.

10 Dicker L, Mosure D, Steece R, Stone K: Laboratory tests used in US public health laboratories for sexually transmitted diseases, 2000. Sex Transm Dis 2004;31:259–264.

11 Yee E, Satterwhite CL, Braxton J, Tran A, Steece R, Weinstock H: Current STD laboratory testing and volume in the United States among public health laboratories, 2007. Presented at 18th ISSTDR (International Society for STD Research), London, 28 June to 7 July, 2009.

12 Dicker LW, Mosure DJ, Levine WC, Black CM, Berman SM: Impact of switching laboratory tests on reported trends in chlamydia trachomatis infections. Am J Epidemiol 2000;151:430–435.

13 Satterwhite CL, Tian LH, Braxton J, Weinstock H: Chlamydia prevalence among women and men entering the National Job Training Program: United States, 2003–2007. Sex Transm Dis 2010;37:63–67.

14 US Preventive Services Task Force: Screening for chlamydial infection: Recommendations and rationale. Am J Prev Med 2001;20:90–94.

15 US Preventive Services Task Force: Screening for chlamydial infection: US Preventive Services Task Force recommendation statement. Ann Intern Med 2007;147:128–134.

16 Meyers D, Halvorson H, Luckhaupt S: Screening for chlamydial infection: an evidence update for the US Preventive Services Task Force. Ann Intern Med 2007;147:135–142.

17 Maloney SK, Johnson C: Why screen for chlamydia? An implementation guide for healthcare providers. Washington, Partnership for Prevention, 2008.

18 Centers for Disease Control and Prevention: Chlamydia screening among sexually active young female enrollees of health plans – United States, 2000–2007. MMWR Morb Mortal Wkly Rep 2009; 58:362–365.

19 National Committee for Quality Assurance: The State of Health Care Quality. Washington, National Committee for Quality Assurance, 2010.

20 Miller WC: Epidemiology of chlamydial infection: are we losing ground? Sex Transm Infect 2008;84: 82–86.

21 Datta S, Torrone E, Kruszon-Moran D, Berman S, Johnson R, Satterwhite C, Papp J, Weinstock H: *Chlamydia trachomatis* trends in the United States among persons 14 to 39 years of age, 1999–2008. Sex Transm Dis 2012;39:92–96.

22 Dicker LW, Mosure DJ, Levine WC: Chlamydia positivity versus prevalence: what's the difference? Sex Transm Dis 1998;25:251–253.

23 Satterwhite CL, Datta SD, Weinstock HS, Chlamydia trends in the United States: results from multiple data sources. Presented at 19th International Society for STD Research (ISSTDR), Quebec, 10–13 July, 2011.

24 Satterwhite C, Gray A, Berman S, Weinstock H, Kleinbaum D, Howards P: *Chlamydia trachomatis* infections among women attending prenatal clinics: United States, 2004–2009. Sex Transm Dis 2012;39: 416–420.

25 Mertz KJ, Ransom RL, St Louis ME, Groseclose SL, Hadgu A, Levine WC, Hayman C: Prevalence of genital chlamydial infection in young women entering a national job training program, 1990–1997. Am J Public Health 2001;91:1287–1290.

26 Joesoef MR, Mosure D: Prevalence trends in chlamydial infections among young women entering the National Job Training Program, 1998–2004. Sex Transm Dis 2006;33:571–575.

27 Haggerty C, Gottlieb S, Taylor B, Low N, Xu F, Ness R: Risk of sequelae after *Chlamydia trachomatis* genital infection in women. J Infect Dis 2010; 201(suppl 2):S134–S155.

28 Oakeshott P, Kerry S, Aghaizu A, Atherton H, Hay S, Taylor-Robinson D, Simms I, Hay P: Randomised controlled trial of screening for *Chlamydia trachomatis* to prevent pelvic inflammatory disease: the POPI (prevention of pelvic infection) trial. BMJ 2010;340:c1642–c1642.

29 Paavonen J, Westrom L, Eschenbach D: Pelvic inflammatory disease; in Holmes KK, et al. (eds): Sexually Transmitted Diseases, ed 4. New York, McGraw-Hill, 2008.

30 Wallace LA, Scoular A, Hart G, Reid M, Wilson P, Goldberg DJ: What is the excess risk of infertility in women after genital chlamydia infection? A systematic review of the evidence. Sex Transm Infect 2008;84:171–175.

31 Bohm MK, Newman L, Satterwhite CL, Tao G, Weinstock HS: Pelvic inflammatory disease among privately insured women, United States, 2001–2005. Sex Transm Dis 2009;37:131–136.

32 Hoover K, Tao G, Kent C: Trends in the diagnosis and treatment of ectopic pregnancy in the United States. Obstet Gynecol 2010;115:495–502.

33 Stephen E, Chandra A: Declining estimates of infertility in the United States: 1982–2002. Fertil Steril 2006;86:516–523.

34 Brunham R, Pourbohloul B, Mak S, White R, Rekart M: The unexpected impact of a *Chlamydia trachomatis* infection control program on susceptibility to reinfection. J Infect Dis 2005;192:1836–1844.

35 Gotz H, Lindback J, Ripa T, Arneborn M, Ramsted K, Ekdahl K: Is the increase in notifications of *Chlamydia trachomatis* infections in Sweden the result of changes in prevalence, sampling frequency or diagnostic methods? Scand J Infect Dis 2002;34: 28–34.

36 Low N: Screening programmes for chlamydial infection: when will we ever learn? BMJ 2007;334:725–728.

37 Brunham RC, Rekart ML: The arrested immunity hypothesis and the epidemiology of chlamydia control. Sex Transm Dis 2008;35:53–54.

38 Hillis SD, Joesoef R, Marchbanks PA, Wasserheit JN, Cates W Jr, Westrom L: Delayed care of pelvic inflammatory disease as a risk factor for impaired fertility. Am J Obstet Gynecol 1993;168:1503–1509.

39 Maciosek M, Coffield A, Edwards N, Flottemesch T, Goodman M, Solberg L: Priorities among effective clinical preventive services: results of a systematic review and analysis. Am J Prev Med 2006;31:52–61.

40 Low N: Publication of report on chlamydia control activities in Europe. Euro Surveill 2008;13:18924.

41 Scholes D, Stergachis A, Heidrich FE, Andrilla H, Holmes KK, Stamm WE: Prevention of pelvic inflammatory disease by screening for cervical chlamydial infection. NEJM 1996;334:1362–1366.

42 Ostergaard L, Andersen B, Mller JK, Olesen F: Home sampling versus conventional swab sampling for screening of *Chlamydia trachomatis* in women: a cluster-randomized 1-year follow-up study. Clin Infect Dis 2000;31:951–957.

43 Bloom MS, Hu Z, Gaydos JC, Brundage JF, Tobler SK: Incidence rates of pelvic inflammatory disease diagnoses among Army and Navy recruits and potential impacts of chlamydia screening policies. Am J Prev Med 2008;34:471–477.

44 Clark KL, Howell MR, Li Y, Powers T, McKee KT Jr., Quinn TC, Gaydos JC, Gaydos CA: Hospitalization rates in female US Army recruits associated with a screening program for *Chlamydia trachomatis*. Sex Transm Dis 2002;29:1–5.

45 Egger M, Low N, Smith GD, Lindblom B, Herrmann B: Screening for chlamydial infections and the risk of ectopic pregnancy in a county in Sweden: ecological analysis. BMJ 1998;316:1776–1780.

46 Hillis SD, Nakashima A, Amsterdam L, Pfister J, Vaughn M, Addiss D, Marchbanks PA, Owens LM, Davis JP: The impact of a comprehensive chlamydia prevention program in Wisconsin. Fam Plann Perspect 1995;27:108–111.

47 Kamwendo F, Forslin L, Bodin L, Danielsson D: Epidemiology of ectopic pregnancy during a 28 year period and the role of pelvic inflammatory disease. Sex Transm Infect 2000;76:28–32.

48 Moss NJ, Ahrens K, Kent CK, Klausner JD: The decline in clinical sequelae of genital *Chlamydia trachomatis* infection supports current control strategies. J Infect Dis 2006;193:1336–1338.

49 Sutton M, Sternberg M, Zaidi A, St Louis M, Markowitz L: Trends in pelvic inflammatory disease hospital discharges and ambulatory visits, United States, 1985–2001. Sex Transm Dis 2005;32:778–784.

50 Gottlieb SL, Berman SM, Low N: Screening and treatment to prevent sequelae in women with *Chlamydia trachomatis* genital infection: how much do we know? J Infect Dis 2010;201(suppl 2):S156–S167.

51 Peterman TA, Gottlieb SL, Berman SM: Commentary: *Chlamydia trachomatis* screening: what are we trying to do? Int J Epidemiol 2009;38:449–451.

52 Low N, Hocking J: Republished paper: the POPI trial: What does it mean for chlamydia control now? Postgrad Med J 2010;86:571–572.

53 Nguyen TQ, Ford CA, Kaufman JS, Leone PA, Suchindran C, Miller WC: Infrequent chlamydial testing among young adults: financial and regional differences. Sex Transm Dis 2008;35:725–730.

54 Heijne JC, Tao G, Kent CK, Low N: Uptake of regular chlamydia testing by US women: a longitudinal study. Am J Prev Med 2010;39:243–250.

55 Friedman AL, Bloodgood B: 'Something we'd rather not talk about': findings from CDC exploratory research on sexually transmitted disease communication with girls and women. J Womens Health (Larchmt) 2010;19:1823–1831.

56 McFarlane M: GYT evaluation (part II). Presented at 2010 National STD Prevention Conference, Atlanta, 8–11 March, 2010.

57 Gift T, Gaydos C, Kent C, Marrazzo J, Rietmeijer C, Schillinger J, Dunne E: The program cost and cost-effectiveness of screening men for chlamydia to prevent pelvic inflammatory disease in women. Sex Transm Dis 2008;35:S66–S75.

58 Dunne EF, Chapin JB, Rietmeijer CA, Kent CK, Ellen JM, Gaydos CA, Willard NJ, Kohn R, Lloyd L, Thomas S, Birkjukow N, Chung S, Klausner J, Schillinger JA, Markowitz LE: Rate and predictors of repeat *Chlamydia trachomatis* infection among men. Sex Transm Dis 2008;35:S40–S44.

59 Hosenfeld C, Workowski K, Berman S, Zaidi A, Dyson J, Mosure D, Bolan G, Bauer H: Repeat infection with chlamydia and gonorrhea among females: a systematic review of the literature. Sex Transm Dis 2009;36:478–489.

60 Paneth-Pollak R, Schillinger JA, Borrelli JM, Handel S, Pathela P, Blank AS: Using STD electronic medical record data to drive public health program decisions in New York City. Am J Public Health 2010;100:586–590.

61 Kretzschmar M, Satterwhite C, Leichliter J, Berman S: Effects of screening and partner notification on chlamydia prevalence in the United States: a modeling study. Sex Transm Dis 2012;39:325–331.

62 Golden MR, Hogben M, Handsfield HH, St Lawrence JS, Potterat JJ, Holmes KK: Partner notification for HIV and STD in the United States: low coverage for gonorrhea, chlamydial infection, and HIV. Sex Transm Dis 2003;30:490–496.

63 Centers for Disease Control and Prevention: Expedited partner therapy in the management of sexually transmitted diseases. Atlanta, US Department of Health and Human Services. 2006.

64 Trelle S, Shang A, Nartey L, Cassell JA, Low N: Improved effectiveness of partner notification for patients with sexually transmitted infections: systematic review. BMJ 2007;334:354.

65 Centers for Disease Control and Prevention: Chlamydia prevention: challenges and strategies for reducing disease burden and sequelae. MMWR Morb Mortal Wkly Rep 2011;60:370–373.

66 US Preventive Services Task Force: Behavioral counseling to prevent sexually transmitted infections: US Preventive Services Task Force recommendation statement. Ann Intern Med 2008;149:491–496.

67 Ness RB, Randall H, Richter HE, Peipert JF, Montagno A, Soper DE, Sweet RL, Nelson DB, Schubeck D, Hendrix SL, Bass DC, Kip KE: Condom use and the risk of recurrent pelvic inflammatory disease, chronic pelvic pain, or infertility following an episode of pelvic inflammatory disease. Am J Public Health 2004;94:1327–1329.

68 Minnis AM, Padian NS: Effectiveness of female controlled barrier methods in preventing sexually transmitted infections and HIV: current evidence and future research directions. Sex Transm Infect 2005;81:193–200.

69 Turner AN, Morrison CS, Padian NS, Kaufman JS, Behets FM, Salata RA, Mmiro FA, Chipato T, Celentano DD, Rugpao S, Miller WC: Male circumcision and women's risk of incident chlamydial, gonococcal, and trichomonal infections. Sex Transm Dis 2008;35:689–695.

70 Chandra A, Mosher W, Copen C, Sionean C: Sexual behavior, sexual attraction, and sexual identity in the United States: data from the 2006–2008 National Survey of Family Growth. Natl Health Stat Report 2011;36:1–49.

71 Gottlieb SL, Martin DH, Xu F, Byrne GI, Brunham RC: Summary: the natural history and immunobiology of *Chlamydia trachomatis* genital infection and implications for chlamydia control. J Infect Dis 2010;201(suppl 2):S190–S204.

Catherine Lindsey Satterwhite
Department of Preventive Medicine and Public Health
University of Kansas Medical School
3901 Rainbow Blvd, MS 1008, Kansas City, KS 66160 (USA)
E-Mail csatterwhite@kumc.edu

Satterwhite · Douglas

Chapter 2

Black CM (ed): Chlamydial Infection: A Clinical and Public Health Perspective.
Issues Infect Dis. Basel, Karger, 2013, vol 7, pp 25–60 (DOI: 10.1159/000348751)

Chlamydia trachomatis Pathogenicity and Disease

Deborah Dean

Center for Immunobiology and Vaccine Development, Children's Hospital Oakland Research Institute,
Oakland, Calif., and Department of Bioengineering, University of California at Berkley and San Francisco,
Calif., USA

Abstract

Disease pathogenesis due to *Chlamydia trachomatis* is a complicated process that involves: (1) exposure to the organism and infectivity; (2) survival within the host cell; (3) virulence associated with specific strain types; (4) innate and acquired immunity, and (5) host genetic susceptibility to infection and disease. While antibiotics have been successful in treating most uncomplicated *C. trachomatis* urogenital infections, treatment does not generally resolve persistent infections or prevent autoimmunity as in Reiter's Syndrome, a chronic debilitating reactive arthritis caused by *C. trachomatis* and other bacterial pathogens. Furthermore, the extent of treatment failure is virtually unknown because of the lack of cost-effective point-of-care diagnostics and techniques for unambiguous strain typing before and after treatment. These drawbacks are compounded by the fact that the majority of female and male infections are asymptomatic, which provides an ongoing opportunity for silent transmission and the development of disease. In addition, repeat and persistent infections are common among at risk adolescent and young adult populations. Even with appropriate detection, there is increasing evidence for antibiotic resistance to the common drugs used to treat *C. trachomatis*. Consequently, the inability to adequately prevent, diagnose, treat and eradicate infection provides the opportunity for pathogenicity and disease.

Chlamydia trachomatis is an obligate intracellular Gram-negative organism that is responsible for a broad diversity of diseases among men and women throughout the world. Over 100 million *C. trachomatis* urogenital infections occur each year according to the World Health Organization [1]. In the USA alone, 1.2 million *C. trachomatis* sexually transmitted disease (STD) cases were reported in 2009 [2]. However, the CDC estimates that the rates of infection are actually closer to 2.8 million each year [3]. The fact that the majority of female and male infections are asymptomatic (70 and 50%, respectively) [4] is an important component in increased transmission, infection and disease. The barriers to stemming this epidemic are a lack of: (1) a vaccine; (2) an effective microbicide or mucosal therapy that can prevent *C. trachomatis* transmission, and (3) a rapid point-of-care diagnostic for screening and test-of-cure.

The major outer membrane protein (MOMP) of *C. trachomatis* contains serovar-, subspecies- and species-specific epitopes [5]. Eighteen serological variants (serovars) of *C. trachomatis* have been identified based on monoclonal antibody (MAb) typing of the antigenically diverse MOMP [6], which contains four variable segments (VS) and five constant segments (CS). The serovars are also grouped based on MAb typing patterns: B class (B, Ba, D, Da, E, L2, L2a, L2b); C class (A, C, H, I, Ia, J, Ja, K, L1, L3), and Intermediate class (F, G, Ga). These serovars exhibit a broad range of tissue tropism and invasiveness in the human host. However, the antibody-based classes do not correlate with tissue tropism, invasiveness, phenotypic disease characteristics or disease outcome. The *ompA* gene, which encodes MOMP, has refined strain typing since it varies considerably within serovars [7–15]. *ompA* polymorphisms have been identified in 39–66% of ocular trachoma and STD samples worldwide [7–15] and, in some cases, can distinguish ocular versus genital isolates that represent the same serovar [16]. These data suggest that *ompA* genotyping can identify nearly tenfold more *C. trachomatis* subtypes or strains than serotyping. Consequently, this chapter refers to strains instead of serovars unless the study refers to organisms that were specifically typed by MAbs.

Three multilocus sequencing typing schemes have been developed for *C. trachomatis*. The scheme by Klint et al. [17] does not exclusively use housekeeping genes and, therefore, has limited use in epidemiologic studies. The scheme by Pannekoek et al. [18] has low discriminatory power for differentiating B from lymphogranuloma venereum (LGV) strains. The scheme by Dean et al. [19] differentiates strains by ocular trachoma, LGV and non-LGV sexually transmitted infection disease groups as well as identifying isolates that appear to be recombinants of *C. trachomatis* strains. Single nucleotide polymorphisms (SNPs) that correlate with disease phenotypes were also identified in the latter study. These findings suggest that applying this multilocus sequencing typing approach more broadly will greatly enhance our understanding of diseases for all types of *Chlamydiaceae* infections and will capture outbreak strains that occur from recombination, although ideally whole genome sequencing would provide the best discriminatory power to identify strain types and their disease associations. Indeed, the relatively recent discovery of *Chlamydiaceae* intra- and interspecies recombination [20–27] (rearrangement of DNA sequences within the cell and incorporation of DNA from outside the cell, introduced by lateral gene transfer, respectively) indicates that knowledge of the location and mechanisms of recombination or lateral gene transfer among strains or between species is needed to identify current recombinant strains, understand how new strains emerge and explore their role in disease pathogenesis.

Because of the inability to reliably genetically manipulate *C. trachomatis*, the pathogenic mechanisms of the diseases caused by the organism remain poorly defined. In this chapter, the following topics are covered: (1) exposure to the organism and infectivity of the different serological variants or strains of *C. trachomatis* and their tissue tropism, without which there would be no pathology; (2) how the organism survives inside the cell to replicate, undergo additional rounds of replication or persist to cause acute and chronic disease; (3) the different virulence factors of the organism and how each may be associated with disease pathogenesis; (4) what we know about innate and acquired immunity and their role in infection resolution, persistence and disease; and (5) host genetic susceptibility to infection and disease, a relatively new area of research that will provide complementary insight into disease pathogenesis.

Exposure and Infectivity

Transmission and Repeat Infection
C. trachomatis is an obligate intracellular Gram-negative organism that is transmitted by intimate direct sexual contact between mucosal surfaces or by hand to mucosal to hand to mucosal inoculation. Currently, because of the high prevalence of asymptomatic infections, these individuals are unlikely to seek treatment and, therefore, represent a significant reservoir for ongoing transmission of the organism. Indeed, 40% of women with untreated infection will develop pelvic inflammatory disease (PID), 20% of whom will become infertile, 18% will experience debilitating chronic pelvic pain and 9% will have a life-threatening ectopic pregnancy [4, 28, 29]. PID can be self-limiting, yet, in many cases, fallopian tube and extraluminal scarring are the sequelae of these infections [30]. If an infected pregnant woman is not treated, her baby has a 50% chance of developing conjunctivitis and a 20% chance of pneumonitis in the first 6 months of life [31, 32]. *C. trachomatis* is also a risk factor for invasive squamous-cell carcinoma of the cervix [33–35] and a complicating factor in HIV-1 infection and transmission [36–38]. Men can develop epididymitis and prostatitis [reviewed in Cunningham and Beagley, 39], and, among men who have sex with men (MSM), severe proctitis [30]. There are no studies that have evaluated screening for *C. trachomatis*, especially in asymptomatic populations, and the effect on sequelae such as PID, tubal inflammation or tubal factor infertility (TFI) [40]. However, in a study by Jones et al. [41], asymptomatic women who were at risk for STDs were found to have endometrial *C. trachomatis* infections in 41% of the cases.

Repeat- [42–47] and mixed-strain [7, 15, 48–51] infections are a common occurrence among at risk populations, including adolescents, young adults, commercial sex workers and their partners. Studies in Finland and the USA have found that a prior documented chlamydial infection was a risk factor for recurrent infections [52, 53]. Reinfection has been reported months to a year or so after infection at rates as high as 59.6% [44, 45, 54–56], despite appropriate treatment [57, 58]. Reinfection occurs partly because immunity to the initial infection is short-lived [reviewed in Batteiger et al., 43] and is serovar specific, although infection with different serovars over time is thought to induce longer-term immunity across serovars [50]. In a study that evaluated organism load by quantitative DNA methods, there was a significantly lower load of organisms with each repeat infection that was not associated with *ompA* genotype, suggesting that immunity was not serovar specific, but that perhaps immunity limited replication [59]. Furthermore, antibiotic treatment may increase the risk of reinfection because of the limited time in which the individual has an opportunity to mount an immune response. This concept is supported by studies in both STD [60] and trachoma [61] patients as well as in the murine model of chlamydial genital tract infections [62]. In the latter case, immunity was attenuated if antibiotics were given prior to induction of a protective immune response.

Studies of salpingitis, ectopic pregnancy and ocular trachoma in animal models as well as the few studies involving humans suggest that recurrent, rather than primary, infection is responsible for the scarring that leads to the sequelae of tubal infertility and ectopic pregnancy [7, 47, 63–67]. Unfortunately, there are few studies that have evaluated initial or repeat lower genital tract or tubal infections and their association with infertility or ectopic pregnancy [68]. In one study, women with two or more chlamydial infections were shown to be at a significant 4.5- to 6.4-fold increased risk of PID and a 2- to 4.5-fold increased risk for ectopic pregnancy [67]. Epidemiologic analyses have also found that there is an association between prior *C. trachomatis* infections of the fallopian tubes and ectopic pregnancies [69]. These studies are supported by research in the macaque model of upper genital tract infections where repeated but not primary infection was required for the complications of tubal and periadnexal scarring, salpingitis and perihepatitis [70]. Finally, race, coinfection with concurrent gonorrhea, and past history of STDs are also important factors associated with recurrent chlamydial infections [71]. The data from these as well as other studies suggest that progression of disease is associated with an immunopathogenic response that occurs following repeat infection [reviewed in Carey and Beagley, 63]. The role of mixed infections in disease pathogenesis is not known.

Attachment and Tissue Tropism
While many eukaryotic cells are susceptible to infection, such as monocytes, macrophages, endometrial cells, endothelial cells and dendritic cells, epithelial cells of the urogenital tract and, in particular, the columnar epithelia of the endocervix are the primary target and point of entry for the organism. Cervical ectopy that exposes more of the columnar epithelium in adolescent females provides an increased risk for infection [72]. It is not known how many organisms are required to cause infection nor the mechanism(s) or rate by which *C. trachomatis* spreads from the lower to the upper genital tract. In the murine model of chlamydial STDs, both the dose and rate at which ascension occurs have been evaluated [73–75]. Interestingly, dose does appear to affect infection in different strains of mice [76] and also ascension to the upper genital tract but does not appear to alter the sequelae of hydrosalpinx and cellular pathology [73]. Whether this is applicable to humans is not known.

The extracellular elementary body (EB) is the infectious form of the organism. For attachment to the host cell, a number of ligands have been proposed that include the MOMP, glycosaminoglycan (GAG), OmcB, PmpD and a high-mannose oligosaccharide glycan moiety [reviewed in Cocchiaro and Valdivia, 77]. The proposed cellular receptors are the estrogen receptor, heparan sulfate receptor and mannose and mannose 6-P receptors [78, 79]. Interestingly, competitive inhibition of attachment has been documented for heterologous serovars of the organism [80]. Recently, protein disulfide isomerase (PDI) has been implicated in attachment given new data that PDI-deficient cells are not efficiently invaded by *C. trachomatis* [81]. The translocated actin-recruiting phosphoprotein (TARP) binds to and nucleates actin, which is essential for EB invasion of the cell [82]. Both TARP and CT694 are bacterial proteins that are translocated into the cell cytoplasm at attachment and play a role in actin remodeling and cytoskeleton rearrangement, which facilitates movement of the EB into the cell and formation of a phagosome, termed an inclusion, that surrounds the organism during its developmental cycle. Recent data suggest that mutations in TARP among strains that are responsible for the same disease (e.g. strains E and F associated with cervicitis) may be involved in niche-specific adaptation in the host [83] (see 'Virulence Factors', below).

There are other examples of tissue tropism specificity for adherence of *C. trachomatis*. The ocular strains A, B, Ba and C are responsible for a chronic inflammatory disease of the conjunctivae, termed trachoma, which is the leading cause of preventable blindness in the world today [84]. All except strain A have been recovered from the urogenital tract. While the ocular strains are not considered to play a role in upper genital tract pathology, recent data suggests that these strains may be responsible for reactive arthritis as they have been identified by PCR in synovial tissue of individuals so afflicted [85]. In both murine and rat models, metabolically active C, E and K strains were found in the joints after vaginal infection [86]. Chlamydial DNA has also been identified in the sacroiliac joint [87]. A potential explanation for these findings is that cells infected with ocular strains may disseminate more efficiently from the primary site of infection to the joints than urogenital strains [88], although appropriate studies are needed to advance this hypothesis. The initial urogenital infection elicits an inflammatory response, attracting mononuclear cells that may become infected and subsequently transport the organism via the circulation to the synovium [89]. However, it is not understood whether there is a particular homing to the joints or whether microvascular damage facilitates migration of the monocytes into the tissue. It is also not clear why only a small fraction of patients develop reactive arthritis and why approximately 50% of these individuals progress to chronic disease [87]. Importantly, *C. trachomatis* appears to reside within monocytes or macrophages of the synovium [90–92] for extended periods in a persistent state, a common survival mechanism exploited by the organism [93]. There is also evidence that *Chlamydia pneumoniae* may similarly be a trigger for reactive arthritis [94–96]. The pathologic features include invasion of the joint by polymorphonuclear leukocytes in addition to plasma cell infiltration. While the joint is not usually eroded as in rheumatoid arthritis, fibrin deposition is present throughout the tissue, and the presence of other proteinaceous substances in the walls of the vasculature are responsible for microvascular occlusion and congestion. It has been suggested that eradication of the organism from the joints might be able to prevent the progression of these sequelae [86]. Finally, some recent data indicate that strains Ba and C that are recovered from the urogenital tract are actually genetically distinct from those causing trachoma [Dean et al., unpubl. data]. If this is borne out by additional genetic and genomic studies, it would support the notion that there are actually distinct urogenital and ocular strains (i.e. urogenital Ba and C strains distinct from ocular Ba and C strains) that exhibit selective tissue tropism.

The majority of STDs are caused by strains D through K, Da, Ga, Ia and Ja. They preferentially infect the urethral, rectal and cervical mucosal epithelia. However, these strains also infect the conjunctiva, often producing a self-limiting infection that rarely causes disease. *ompA* genotyping studies have found that certain variant strains of F are associated with upper genital tract infection compared with cervical infection where strain E was found to predominate [15]. No correlation has been documented between strain or degree of inflammation for urethral and cervical samples [49]. Another study noted that recurrent infections with the same serovar were common among patients with concurrent gonorrhea but no specific serovar was a risk factor for coinfection [97]. The pathology of women with upper genital tract infections is also probably not restricted to specific strains, although there is a shortage of studies in this area, and is characterized by lymphocyte and plasma cell infiltration of the stromal layer and polymorphonuclear cells localized to the epithelial layer [98]. Importantly, strains D, G and J are also prevalent in anorectal infections unlike other urogenital strains [99–102] except for L1, L2, L2a, L2b and L3 [103]. The latter comprise the LGV biologic variants (biovars) of *C. trachomatis* that are responsible for more invasive disease.

The LGV strains do not appear to have specific tropism as they are able to infect any mucosal site but, unlike the other urogenital strains, they can invade the basal layers and disseminate via regional lymphatics to draining lymph nodes. Consequently, the LGV strains are associated with inguinal syndromes including regional lymphadenitis, inguinal buboes and bubonulus. Recently, sporadic and ongoing outbreaks of LGV among MSM have been documented in Australia, Europe and the USA [104–107]. A curious feature of the clinical presentation is a lack of the inguinal syndrome [107]. There have also been reports of LGV outbreak strains (e.g. L2b) [108]. This suggests the emergence of new strains that may possess different virulence factors to limit dissemination but that are still capable of causing severe localized mucosal disease. Indeed, a recent study [24] discovered a variant strain of L2, termed L2c, that was isolated from an MSM and contains a functional toxin gene, which was likely acquired from a D strain by recombination. It is probable that the toxin limits invasion and lymphatic spread due to local cytotoxicity (discussed in 'Virulence Factors', below). The primary pathogenic process in LGV is proliferation of endothelial cells of the lymphatic and lymph node vessels. Areas of necrosis form within the nodes, attracting polymorphonuclear leukocytes with the eventual formation of buboes, fistulas and sinus tracts. The healing process occurs by fibrosis, which ablates the normal vessels leading to induration, edema and restriction of the blood supply that can result in ulceration. A similar process takes place in the rectal mucosa with inflammation and the formation of strictures and fistulae to adjacent anatomic sites. It has been postulated that the tissue damage is associated with cell-mediated hypersensitivity to the organism, possibly from organism persistence or reinfection [109]. Both are considered important in the fibrosis seen in upper genital tract infections [98] and trachoma [110]. In addition, host immunity is thought to limit the spread of the organism but does not eliminate it. Indeed, *C. trachomatis* has been isolated from inguinal buboes that first occurred 20 years earlier [111]. LGV strains can also spread via the blood stream to cause disease at more distant sites such as meningitis [112] and reactive arthritis [113]. The molecular mechanisms for dissemination and fibrosis formation remain unknown.

Survival within the Host Cell

Inclusion Formation and Expansion, and Effector Proteins
C. trachomatis must infect a host cell in order to replicate. And the intracellular nature of infection affords the organism some protection from annihilation by the host. As mentioned above, the organism has a biphasic developmental cycle that begins when the EB comes in contact with the host cell and is taken into the cell either by endophagocytosis, pinocytosis or receptor-mediated endocytosis. The organism somehow prevents routing into the lysosomal pathway [114], which circumvents destruction and allows replication to proceed. Nucleoid decondensation occurs as the EB differentiates into the metabolically active, noninfectious reticulate body (RB) and, within 15 min, bacterial proteins are produced using its own stores of ATP and essential phosphate compounds, metabolites [115] and other host cell substrates (e.g. nucleotides, amino acids, sphingolipids, cholesterol and glycerophospholipids) that are essential for development [reviewed in Saka and Valdivia, 116]. Interestingly, the LGV strains, unlike all other strains, require methionine while the ocular strains require tryptophan. Nutritional deficiencies, therefore, can affect replication and drive the organism into a persistent state that has pathogenic implications for the host (see 'Virulence Factors', below). A number of cellular organelles are associated with the inclusion but, to date, only species-specific differences have been noted that may affect acquisition of host nutrients and thereby disease pathogenesis, although multiple pathways are likely used by *C. trachomatis* to acquire what it needs for replication and survival [reviewed in Cocchiaro and Valdivia, 77]. Mechanisms for transfer of nutrients across the inclusion membrane have not been elucidated, although there is evidence that the inclusion is porous to low molecular weight, uncharged, molecules [117].

 C. trachomatis possesses a type III secretion system (T3SS), similar to those found in other Gram-negative bacteria, which is considered a virulence determinant and functions by secreting proteins into the host cell to favorably modulate the intracellular environment for development. Surface projections on the EB and RB have been observed by electron microscopy that may represent the T3SS [118]. *C. trachomatis* secrete proteins prior to invasion of the host cell and once inside the cell. The EB contains the components of the T3SS and secretes TARP outside the cell [119], which is essential for cell invasion, as discussed above. Within 1–3 h inside the cell, secreted proteins transform the plasma membrane derived phagosome into an inclusion comprised primarily of chlamydial inclusion membrane proteins [120]; other proteins localized in proximity to the inclusion or secreted into the cytosol include CopN, Cap1, CADD, CT620, CT621, CT711 and nuclear effector protein [119, 121–125]. Interestingly, the T3SS is not the only system for secretion of effector proteins. The chlamydial protease/proteasome-like activity factor (CPAF) is secreted into the cytosol by Sec-dependent transport [126]. While secreted effector proteins are largely considered species-specific, there are few data describing genetic variants of these proteins among different strains of *C. trachomatis* that may affect invasion, development and evasion of host immunity with a consequent impact on disease pathogenesis.

As replication progresses and the inclusion enlarges, F-actin and intermediate filaments create a stable cytoskeletal structure that contain the inclusion. CPAF cleaves the intermediate filaments to allow expansion and stability of the inclusion [127]. Recently it has been shown that sphingolipid biosynthesis is also necessary for integrity of the inclusion [128]. Containment of the inclusion also likely limits activation of the host innate immune response. While the organism secretes proteins to ensure maintenance of the inclusion, it must also ensure that it does not trigger early cell death since a sufficient period of time is needed before releasing viable EBs for the next round of infection. Early apoptosis has recently been shown to result in impaired development of the organism [129]. Thus, inhibition of cellular apoptosis is used to prevent cell death as the inclusion grows. However, it is also used to avoid detection by the host, at least for the duration of its developmental cycle. The effector protein CPAF appears to degrade BH-3-only proteins of the Bcl-2 subfamily members that are responsible for detecting stress signals in the cell and triggering apoptosis [130]. While different antiapoptotic pathways appear to be induced by *C. trachomatis* [reviewed in Cocchiaro and Valdivia, 77], the antiapoptotic Mcl-1 protein activates the signaling cascade of Raf/MEK/ERK that was found to be linked to inflammation via production of the inflammatory cytokine interleukin (IL)-8, although only strain L2 was examined in that study [131]. Thus, not all antiapoptotic pathways are equal in terms of minimizing impact on the host. It is also not clear whether all stains use the same pathways or activate Mdl-1.

Persistence

At some point during development, replication can be arrested with expansion of the RBs to aberrant forms that are in a stationary phase. During this phase, the cell is in a state of persistence where the organism resides within the cell in a viable but noncultivable state. In humans, it is difficult to unequivocally prove that persistent *C. trachomatis* STDs occur because one cannot entirely control for reexposure to untreated partner(s) [132] or recent transmission from an infected trachoma patient. There is also concern about emerging resistance to common antibiotics with the consequence of persistent infection [58, 133–135]. The evidence supporting persistence comes from in vitro systems, animal models and human populations. Induction of persistence is not entirely understood. In vitro studies have shown that *C. trachomatis*-infected HeLa 229 cells develop aberrant inclusion morphology in response to IFN-γ, exposure to penicillin or deprivation of essential amino acids [136, 137]. Inhibition of intracellular growth by IFN-γ is achieved by depletion of tryptophan, which occurs by induction of the tryptophan-degrading enzyme, indoleamine dioxygenase, although it is not known if this occurs in vivo. Removal of IFN-γ or penicillin, or replacement of amino acids results in resumption of normal development, including surface protein expression. The addition of tryptophan to the tissue culture also reverses the effects of IFN-γ [138]. Thus, persistence may be widely present among individuals who are culture negative and have clinically unapparent infection. This may be a source for reinfection or spread of infection when environmental or host conditions favor the transformation of the latent form into an infectious or metabolically active one.

Persistence has also been demonstrated in animal models of *C. trachomatis* infection [76, 139–142]. In a murine model of cervical infections, persistent *C. trachomatis* forms were observed by electron microscopy in epithelial cells months after the initial infection [141]. Similarly, apparent clearing of the primary infection was followed by *C. trachomatis* shedding after immunosuppression with cyclophosphamide or cortisone acetate, suggesting that viable organisms were present for at least 4–5 weeks in the mouse genital tract [76]. In the macaque model of salpingitis, persistent *C. trachomatis* DNA and antigens were found in upper genital tract tissue long after treatment was completed [140]. Among STD populations, persistent cervical infections have also been documented [143, 144]. In one study, women with ≥3 *C. trachomatis* recurrences over 2–5 years were found to have same-serovar infections in 24% of the cases [144]. Interestingly, the recurrent serovars were the least common among the population sampled. In the same study, many intervening culture-negative samples were positive by nucleic amplification tests long after residual DNA should have been cleared after treatment, which lends support to the growing body of evidence that *C. trachomatis* organisms persist. These cumulative findings, then, support the notion that *C. trachomatis* may contain specific biologic properties that allow for initial infection and then persistence through modulation of MOMP or other surface-expressed proteins in response to immune or antimicrobial selection. During persistence, there is reduced expression of lipopolysaccharide (LPS) and MOMP but normal or increased expression of *C. trachomatis* heat shock protein 60 (cHSP60) [145]. cHSP60 is considered a virulence factor that induces an adverse immune response associated with pathogenicity in the urogenital tract (discussed in 'Immune Response', below).

Release of Elementary Bodies from the Cell for the Next Round of Replication
Once the developmental cycle is completed, the mature EBs are released by two different mechanisms. One involves cell lysis from protease digestion, which kills the cell. In this scenario, the entire contents of the inclusion are released. The alternative is exocytosis of the intact inclusion without cell death. In one study, a lysosome-mediated repair process was identified that may ensure cell survival in the latter case [146]. Notably, viable bacteria in that study were retained within the host cell, indicating a unique mechanism for ongoing infection and possibly persistence. However, it is not known to what extent cells that have been infected, and where the inclusion has been released, undergo apoptosis or necrosis and what triggers these events. The distinction is important because necrosis tends to elicit an unwanted inflammatory response while apoptosis does not because the contents of the cell remain in an apoptotic body (while the cell undergoes death), which is released and endophagocytosed by other cells [147]. In necrosis, both pathogen and host cell molecules are released that are 'danger signals' for the host. From the pathogen, these include LPS and pathogen-associated molecular molecules (PAMPs) and, from the cell, chromosomal proteins, heat-shock proteins and ATP, to name a few. These mediators induce an inflammatory response that can lead to fibrosis and disease (discussed in 'Immune Response', below). For example, high-mobility group box 1 protein is released when cells undergo necrosis but not apoptosis and is known to mediate inflammation [148]. Poly(ADP-ribose) polymerase 1 repairs DNA and regulates high-mobility group box 1 translocation [149]. In *C. trachomatis* infection, both are degraded [150], suggesting a mechanism for reducing the ensuing inflammation that can occur when cells are damaged during release of the inclusion. The relative frequency of apoptosis versus necrosis that occurs in the host is not known. But, the implications for the host are tremendous and represent an area for further research.

Virulence Factors

Knowledge from Proteomics, Genetics and Genomics
Virulence factors fall into various classifications. They include: (1) adherence and invasion factors that assist bacteria in adhering to and gaining access to host cells (discussed above) – the latter are usually encoded on the chromosome but can be on a plasmid or plasmids; (2) exotoxins are proteins produced and often secreted by bacteria that include enzymes and protein toxins that have various effects on the host cell and tissue; (3) endotoxins are surface proteins such as LPS that can interact with the host cell and may function as adhesins; (4) siderophores that bacteria use to bind host iron for use in their own metabolism; and (5) capsules, which are used to evade phagocytosis and opsonization. Over the last 2 decades there has been accumulated knowledge from proteomics, genetics and genomes regarding chlamydial virulence factors.

While *C. trachomatis* does not possess all of these factors, or at least they have not been described for *Chlamydia*, there are some proteins that fit or somewhat fit within the first three categories.

Major Outer Membrane Protein
The MOMP comprises 60% of the mass of the outer membrane and has been a major focus of research as it contains important neutralizing determinants [151–154], elicits T cell help for antibody production [155] and is involved in T cell immunity [156, 157], contains serovar-, subspecies- and species-specific epitopes [5] and may play a role in attachment and invasion of host cells and in tissue tropism. Thus, MOMP has been, in total or in part, the primary candidate for a chlamydial vaccine. But, *ompA*, which encodes MOMP, is under two types of evolutionary pressure. A number of studies have documented that *ompA* divergence is under selective immune and antibiotic pressure [15, 21, 144]. This is supported by the fact that over 90% of nucleotide substitutions encode amino acid changes in MOMP [7–15] and these changes tend to occur in the same position in both VSs and CSs [16, 158]. One or two amino acid changes are sufficient for immune specificity [6, 9, 159], yet a single change does not guarantee a specificity change [160]. *ompA* diversity may specify slightly different proteins that alter antibody interactions and allow for 'escape mutants' to avoid host immune surveillance [152]. In one in vitro study [161], neutralizing antibodies prevented infection by reference strains, but closely related *ompA* variants escaped neutralization. Thus, variants appear to arise from point mutations from immune pressure.

However, there is also evidence for recombination within *ompA* and in the regions immediately adjacent to the gene that likely occur from mixed or sequential urogenital *C. trachomatis* infections in vivo [20–22, 162]. In the first study to use phylogenetics and statistical modeling of *ompA* for *C. trachomatis* strains, there was significant evidence for intragenic recombination with a high level of recombination relative to substitution processes for the 3′ half of *ompA* [21]. This region contains T cell epitopes, which are important for eliciting protective immunity [155]. The possibility of genetic exchange in a region responsible for immune evasion suggests an opportunity for the organism to continue to evolve strains with better fitness and survival within the host. Furthermore, intra- or intergene recombination that occurs with any frequency could impact on the virulence of the protein. Importantly, genomic uptake of DNA by transformation – a likely mechanism employed by *C. trachomatis* – can occur not just from coinfection, but also from sequential infections, which provides multiple chances for genetic transfer to occur over time. From recent studies, *ompA* is not the only gene that is important for strain evolution and immunomodulation.

Polymorphic Membrane Proteins
The discovery of the nine-member polymorphic membrane protein (Pmp) gene (*pmp*) family in the D strain genome has provided an additional focus for genes that

may be important in *C. trachomatis* biology. This is underscored by the fact that the family is unique to the genus *Chlamydia* and comprises a surprising >7% of the genome, and interspecies amino acid sequence homology is <50% compared to 70–80% for other surface proteins [163]. The Pmps are considered autotransporters and cumulative evidence supports their role as immunogenic proteins. In vitro studies have shown that all *pmp* paralogs are transcribed for *C. trachomatis* [164]. Pmps E, G and H of L2 have been identified as outer membrane proteins that were expressed late in development [165, 166], while more recent studies identified early expression at 2 h for all Pmps [167]. Importantly, immunoglobulins in sera from adolescents infected with strains D, E and G, but not other strains, were shown to be reactive to recombinant PmpC [167]. Subsequent studies support these findings and have shown that patients with urogenital *C. trachomatis* infections have differential systemic antibody responses to one or multiple recombinant Pmps [168, 169]. Indeed, there is considerable sequence variation for *pmps* for reference strains and more recent clinical isolates, including deletions and insertion sequences [22]. There is also evidence for SNPs within some Pmps that correlate with human leukocyte antigen (HLA) class I and II allele T cell epitopes [170]. In this latter study, because of the high number of SNPs in some *pmps* compared to *ompA* and the even higher number of nonsynonymous amino acid mutations in PmpF, this protein was further evaluated. The location of clustered amino acid variation included the central region of the passenger domain, which was found to contain a disproportional number of MHC class II epitopes, suggesting that variation in PmpF may be driven by immune selection. This would certainly be the case if the passenger domain comes in contact with the host cell cytosol where it could be targeted by CD4+ cytotoxic T cells [171].

Gomes et al. [22] was the first to perform phylogenetic analyses of complete *pmp* sequences and found that, for *pmpC*, there was a significant divergence of strains with clustering based on disease phenotypes: trachoma, noninvasive STDs and LGV with one clade including E and F strains, the most common strains among STD populations worldwide. Similar trees for disease phenotype have also been shown for *pmpB*, *pmpF*, *pmpG*, *pmpH* and *pmpI*, but not *pmpA*, *pmpD* or *pmpE* [172, 173]. Furthermore, *pmp* analyses have revealed that urogenital reference strain Da is a recombinant with ocular trachoma strains in the genomic region spanning *pmpE* to *pmpI*, suggesting that acquisition of specific segments of the genome may be beneficial in expanding the range of cellular tropism [168].

Finally, recent investigations have demonstrated that PmpD is an autotransporter component of the bacterial outer membrane [174, 175]. PmpD translocates to the surface of the bacteria, and is likely involved in invasion of the host cell. PmpD appears to function as an adhesin since antibodies raised against the protein were able to block *C. trachomatis* infection of HeLa cells [176]. In the same study, recombinant PmpD was shown to activate human monocytes in vitro and induce the release of IL-8, which is important in the innate immune response.

PorB
PorB is a surface-exposed, outer membrane porin with weak similarity to MOMP. In addition to functioning as a porin, immunoreactive PorB antigens appear to be surface exposed and elicit neutralizing antibodies [177]. There is some sequence variation for PorB among the 15 reference strains examined to date. Strain D contains a stop codon at nucleotide 977 with a predicted truncation of 15 amino acids [178]. However, the other nonsynonymous mutations have not been mapped, and there are no data for recent clinical isolates that tend to have more variable genomes [23, 24]. This will be an important protein to further examine for potential functional differences.

Translocated Actin-Recruiting Phosphoprotein
TARP, as discussed above, is secreted by EBs via the type III secretion system extracellularly and is injected into the host cell [119, 179]. At the site of internalization of the EB, Tarp is involved in actin binding and nucleation and cytoskeleton rearrangement, which facilitates invasion of the cell [119, 180]. While tyrosine phosphorylation of TARP by src family tyrosine kinases is not required for bacterial entry [181, 182], there are variable numbers of tyrosine repeats and actin-binding sites that are mostly conserved for strains that cause the same disease [83]. This might affect actin recruitment and further cytoskeletal rearrangements once inside the cell that could impair inclusion development or expansion or other functions that have not yet been identified. Phylogenetic analysis of reference strains and numerous clinical isolates suggests that this is one of the few genes that may be involved in determining clinical phenotype [83].

C. trachomatis Heat Shock Protein 60
The cHSP60 is a chaperon that is produced by the organism, exposed on the cell surface and thought to be released from the cell during stress [183]. Because of its likely role in persistence, host immune responses and autoimmunity, this virulence factor is discussed below under 'Immune Response'.

Chlamydial Protease/Proteasome-Like Activity factor
CPAF is discussed under 'Survival Within the Host Cell', above, and 'The Immune Response', below.

The Plasticity Zone
As surprising as it was to identify intra- and intergenomic recombination for *C. trachomatis* given the obligate intracellular nature of the organism, it was equally as surprising when Read et al. [184] identified a ~50-kb region of considerable heterogeneity near the origin of the replication and termination region, which was annotated as a plasticity zone (PZ), a term used in other pathogenic bacteria to reflect rapid genetic rearrangements. PZs arise from horizontal gene transfer by phage, conjugative

transposons or plasmid(s). The mechanism used by *C. trachomatis* remains unknown. However, the implications for the evolution of *Chlamydia* and emergence of new pathogenic strains that are more or less virulent is immense.

Genes within the PZ encode proteins that contribute to pathogen virulence such as adhesins, toxins, invasins, iron uptake systems and others. Analyses of available *C. muridarum*, *C. pneumoniae*, *C. caviae*, *C. abortus*, *C. felis* and *C. trachomatis* genomes have revealed a number of 'niche-specific' genes [170, 185, 186] that likely differentiate divergent host and disease phenotypes observed across these species and within species. For example, for *C. trachomatis*, many strains lack a complete toxin gene but contain truncated open reading frames matching N- and C-terminal regions. In vitro studies have shown enhanced cytotoxicity for *C. trachomatis* strains (H and J) that contain the complete gene [187, 188]. This increased cytotoxicity likely limits the degree of dissemination of the organism – *C. trachomatis* LGV and *C. pneumoniae* lack the toxin and are not mucosally restricted, spreading via lymphatics and blood, respectively, in infected carrier cells. A recent study identified a partial, yet functional, toxin gene acquired by an LGV strain that was similar in sequence to strain D [24]. Since no other LGV strains to date are known to contain a complete or partial toxin gene, this suggests that the partial toxin was acquired from a D strain. D strains are prevalent among rectal infections among MSM [100]. The variant LGV strain, referred to as L2c, was isolated from an MSM who presented with severe hemorrhagic proctitis. The lack of an inguinal syndrome in this patient suggested that the toxin may have limited systemic spread of the organism. Indeed, in tissue culture, the strain was far more cytotoxic than other LGV strains. Interestingly, recent data show that the *Chlamydia* toxin indirectly facilitates intracellular growth by damaging host cell actin microfilaments, which would then allow inclusion expansion [189, 190]. It has also been suggested that the toxin inactivates GTPase early in infection when EB(s) are entering the cell, which could assist in thwarting the innate immune response [191, 192]. This is likely just the beginning of our understanding into how this cytotoxin contributes to the invasive properties, variation in tissue tropism, and disease severity and outcome for different strains.

The PZ also contains genes encoding a partial tryptophan biosynthesis operon (*trpR*, *trpB* and *trpA*) and *trpC* (no *trpD* or *trpE*) in *C. trachomatis*, which is missing in *C. muridarum* and *C. abortus*. IFN-γ indirectly depletes tryptophan by activating indoleamine 2,3-dioxygenase that targets intracellular tryptophan [193], an amino acid required for chlamydial replication. Ocular strains lack a functional tryptophan synthase (unlike urogenic strains) due to a frame shift mutation in *trpA* [138, 194, 195]. Consequently, different *C. trachomatis* strains may or may not be able to scavenge host substrates such as indole or other precursors from organisms found in the lower genital tract or use other as yet unidentified enzymes critical for tryptophan biosynthesis. Importantly, the repressor gene functions by responding to changes in tryptophan concentration [196]. Functional differences in the operon, then, would impart a differential susceptibility to IFN-γ that likely correlates with tissue tropism and pathogenicity [138, 191, 194]. As tryptophan is exhausted, the ocular strains may morph into a persistent state while other strains with a functional operon may not, which would explain the earlier findings of a lack of inducible persistence for L2 [197, 198]. However, persistence would also be likely for urogenital strains that reach the upper genital tract where there is no source for indole. Somboonna and Dean [unpubl. data] have recently identified a number of urogenital clinical isolates with mutations in *trpA* that are similar to those in the ocular strains in addition to mutations in *trpB*. These strains were unable to synthesize tryptophan. Thus, mutations in specific *trp* genes or loss of these genes may be necessary for adapting to new host sites of infection and for persistence with the ensuing pathological consequences.

Finally, a few years ago a major discovery was made of four genomic islands carrying tetracycline-resistance plasmids in *C. suis*, a closely related species of *C. trachomatis* [199]. Tetracycline has been broadly used in animal feed to prevent microbial infections. Three islands contained an insertion sequence homologous to *Helicobacter pylori* IS605, suggesting acquisition of the islands from this gut pathogen. Each island is located in the *C. suis* invasion-like gene between the ribosomal operons with insertion likely occurring via a transposase [200]. Even though *C. trachomatis* is not known to contain an invasin gene, this transfer event is worrisome because it suggests the real possibility of this occurring in *C. trachomatis*, especially with the ongoing mass treatment trails for trachoma and the empiric therapy that is used for STDs. This discovery also suggests the need for expansive genome sequencing of hundreds of *C. trachomatis* strains to better understand the potential for acquisition of antibiotic-resistance transposons that would greatly impact pathogenicity and disease.

In sum, the data suggest a role for both MOMP and Pmps in antigenic variation and adaptation to the host environment through selective mutational and recombinant events of their respective genes. Furthermore, MOMP, some Pmps, PorB and TARP are virulence factors involved in tissue tropism and the pathogenesis of early infection. cHSP60 is a virulence factor that elicits a deleterious immune response during persistence and later in infection, while CPAF is critical for maintenance of the inclusion during development. The toxin likely plays a role in infection and tissue tropism but may limit dissemination while causing more severe pathology in the local mucosa. The partial tryptophan operon correlates with tissue tropism and is likely involved in persistence and disease later in infection.

The Immune Response

C. trachomatis attempts to evade the immune response during entry and survival within the host cell as described above. CPAF has been shown to degrade transcription factors such as regulatory factor (RF)X5 [201] and upstream stimulation factor (USF)1 [202], which are required for activation of antigen expression via the major histocompatibility complex. This may aid in chlamydial evasion of host immune recognition. However, higher serum antibody titers against CPAF compared to titers against MOMP or cHSP60 have been detected among women with cervical *C. trachomatis* infections [203], and sera from these same women were shown to neutralize the proteolytic activity of CPAF [204], suggesting an important host mechanism to ensure recognition of pathogen invasion. A recent study showed that CPAF cleaves p65/RelA, which decreases the cell's sensitivity to proinflammatory cytokines, and this event likely promotes intracellular survival of the organism [205].

It is generally accepted that during the initial infection an immune response is elicited, and that both a humeral and protective cell-mediated immune responses are required for infection clearance. Various cells express Toll-like receptors (TLRs) and other pathogen recognition receptors that can recognize specific PAMPs. PAMPs include bacterial DNA and bacterial wall components such as LPS, peptidoglycan and lipoproteins. *C. trachomatis* expresses several cell wall and outer membrane components (discussed above) that may be recognized as PAMPs by TLRs. *C. trachomatis* has recently been found to induce the inflammasome, which is an important component of the innate immune response to protect the host against invading pathogens [reviewed in Abdul-Sater et al., 206]. *C. trachomatis* PAMPs bind to PRR and stimulate intracellular production of various proinflammatory mediators in their immature form. A secondary 'danger signal' in the infected cell, for example, stimulates release of host-cell molecules that induce formation within the cell of an inflammasome, which is a large complex comprised of caspase-1, ASC (an adaptor protein) and Nod-like receptor proteins (NLRP; NLRP3 for *C. trachomatis*). The host immune system differentiates a nonpathogen from a pathogen in that, with a pathogen, there is secretion of IL-1b and IL-18 – inflammasome-dependent caspase-1 activation is required for processing of pro-IL-1b and pro-IL-18 molecules into mature molecules that are subsequently secreted by the cell. *C. trachomatis* has recently been shown to cause potassium efflux and production of radical oxygen species within the cell, which stimulates NLRP3 inflammasome-dependent caspase-1 activation [207]. Interestingly, epithelial cells infected with chlamydiae produce little IL-1b; the majority is produced by monocyte/macrophages and neutrophils [208]. It has also recently been discovered that *C. trachomatis* activation of capase-1 is essential for *C. trachomatis* growth and survival in epithelial cells [207]. Thus, there appears to be a fine balance between the capase-1 induction of the inflammasome and the requirements of capase-1 for *C. trachomatis* survival.

Various *C. trachomatis* PAMPs engage urogenital epithelial cell TLRs, which leads to the production of biologically active mediators such as antimicrobial peptides, proinflammatory cytokines and chemokines, including IL-1, IL-6, IL-8, IL-12 and granulocyte-macrophage colony-stimulating factor [209, 210]. The innate immune cells that are recruited and activated include neutrophils, dendritic cells, macrophages and natural killer cells that stimulate production of IFN-γ and TNF-α that can act to resolve infection [211]. In the macaque 'pocket' model of fallopian tube tissue, the acute infection has been characterized as eliciting a T helper 1 (Th1)-type response that includes IL-2 and IFN-γ but no IL-4 production [212]. More recent studies in women have shown that elevated expression of IL-10, IL-12 and IFN-γ were associated with endocervical infection [213], while lower levels of IL-2 but elevated levels of IL-12 were identified among infected women in another study [214]. In the murine and guinea pig models, there is evidence for similar Th1 cytokine responses involving IFN-γ and production of neutralizing IgG antibodies that are thought to resolve primary infection and protect against reinfection for a few months [reviewed in Rank and Whittum-Hudson, 215]. In addition, there is evidence that presence in the genital tract of CD4+ T lymphocytes that produce IFN-γ is directly related to infection with lower cell counts as clearance of the organism occurs [216–219]. In a rat model of reactive arthritis, higher levels of IFN-γ and TNF-α expression in the synovial tissue were associated with clearance of infection with an expected inverse correlation with synovial weight, which indicated fewer inflammatory cell infiltrations and less edema [220]. Interestingly, there is some evidence that humans will clear their infection without antibiotics over months to years [reviewed in Geisler, 221].

Pathogenic Immune Responses
If resolution of the infection does not occur, however, the inflammatory mediators can participate in tissue destruction and a pathogenic immune response [209, 222]. A recent study of an ex vivo model of human fallopian tubes reported that IL-1 is directly responsible for destruction of ciliated epithelial cells of the fallopian tubes [209]. In another study, cervical cells from women with fertility disorders were stimulated with EBs and found to produce higher levels of IL-1β, IL-6, IL-8 and IL-10 compared with higher levels of IFN-γ and IL-12 among women without these disorders [223], suggesting that a Th1 response can protect against upper genital tract pathology. In trachoma populations, the proinflammatory cytokines IL-1β and TNFα were significantly associated with trachomatous disease and concurrent *C. trachomatis* infection [224]. Increased levels of the Th3/Tr1 cytokine IL-10 were significantly associated with all trachoma grades, while IL-6 and IL-15 were associated with chronic scarring trachoma and also with concurrent *C. trachomatis* infections. While there is some overlap, there are also distinct differences in the immune response. However, in the subcutaneous 'pocket' model of autologous salpingeal tissue from macaques, Th1 cytokines and CD8+ T cell lymphocytes predominated and were associated with tubal fibrosis and scarring after repeated infection [225]. Interestingly, repeat infection in the pocket model resulted in a more rapid infiltration of the fallopian tube tissue by a higher number of lymphocytes (despite a similar inflammatory response in acute infection), follical formation and destruction of the epithelium [65]. These findings were similar to what was found in the guinea pig model using the GPIC agent of *C. caviae* [226]. Reinfection in the guinea pig was also found to correlate with higher levels of oviduct B and T cells but no or few organisms at this site [226], indicating that pathology may be driven by the immune response. In the murine model of chlamyd-

ial genital tract infection, TLR-2 but not TLR-4 was found to be essential for developing upper genital tract pathology [227].

While it has been suggested that the pocket model may not represent what happens in humans because the inoculum is placed directly on the tissue instead of having to travel from the cervix to upper genital tract tissue, studies of the pathology associated with the upper genital tract in women [98] bear close resemblance to that of trachoma. Among trachoma populations, there is direct repeat infection of the conjunctiva. The histopathology of experimental trachoma in cynomolgus monkeys [228] has shown that inflammatory cells in the conjunctivae following reinfection were predominantly plasma cells. There was also development of lymphoid follicles with conjunctival epithelial thinning and, later, patchy areas of degenerating epithelial cells. Leukocytes, B cells and T cells were present in the center of characteristic follicles. Macrophages were also found in this center, which may assist in presentation of antigen to T cells that are then capable of evoking a deleterious immune response. Important structural and functional changes involved disruption of the surface membrane of goblet cells and flattening of microvilli that are part of the normal absorptive surface of the epithelium, which may lead to breakdown of the normal defense mechanism of the epithelium. Interestingly, inclusions, which are present in active chlamydial infections, were absent in epithelial tissue despite the presence of chlamydial antigens. This study has provided some provocative data on immune stimulation and destruction caused by chlamydial antigens as have other studies that have addressed cell mediated immunity [229, 230]. But, ultimately, it is unclear whether these data can be extrapolated to humans. However, for the many asymptomatic chlamydial STIs that do not reach medical attention and for trachoma where treatment is not available, these models seem relevant to what happens in humans since repeat infections are common (see the discussion in 'Transmission and Repeat Infection', above). These data, then, suggest three theories regarding the pathogenesis of sequelae in both the fallopian tubes and conjunctivae: (1) individuals harbor chlamydial organisms that may or may not be in a persistent state, but, provide a continuous or intermittent antigenic stimulus for a deleterious host immune response (which includes the possibility that organisms may be associated with scarring but not causative); this is similar to the cellular paradigm of pathogenesis [reviewed in Darville and Hiltke, 231]; (2) after repeated infection, the organism is eliminated but adaptive immune mediators have been triggered that set up an enhanced inflammatory process (compared to primary infection) with collateral damage that may or may not subside over time and promotes tissue destruction that results in scarring; this is similar to the immunological paradigm of pathogenesis [222], or (3) a combination of both.

Mucosal Immunity in Preventing Recurrent Infection
Mucosal immunity is an important factor in preventing or limiting recurrent *C. trachomatis* infections [232, 233]. IgG responses at the mucosal site are thought to at least partially neutralize the organism and, in concert with memory T cells, partially pre-

vent repeat infection. Previous studies have suggested that the immune responses may protect against reinfection but also facilitate chronic disease [234]. IgA titers in human cervical secretions have been shown to correlate inversely with the number of isolated organisms, suggesting that the mucosal immune response may regulate shedding of *C. trachomatis* [235]. However, IgA and IgG antibodies directed against EBs or cHSP60 have not been found to be associated with protection from repeat infection [236]. In addition, high levels of IFN-γ have also been found in endocervical secretions (and in serum) of women with chlamydial STDs including PID [237, 238] as well as among women with repeat compared to primary infection [239]. While IFN-γ is important for clearing infection, it has also been implicated in induction of persistence, as discussed above. In the murine genital tract model using the *C. muridarum* mouse pneumonitis strain, MoPn, MOMP-specific IgA or IgG MAbs administered vaginally or in serum have been shown to significantly reduce ascending infection and upper genital tract pathology [240]. Immunoglobulin fractions from trachoma patients can also passively neutralize ocular infections in monkeys [241]. sIgA may facilitate bactericidal activity by an interaction with mucosal monocytes, which have been shown to decrease bacterial viability [242], or by enhancing an anti-*C. trachomatis* peroxidase system [243]. Secretory antibodies have been associated with immunity to reinfection in guinea pig eyes [215, 244]. It has also been postulated that the production of IgA1 protease by *Neisseria gonorrhoeae* [245] may reactivate *C. trachomatis*, which could account for the high number of coinfections in STD populations.

Heat Shock Protein 60 and Pathogenicity

There is support in the literature that cHSP60 induces an antigen-specific adaptive response associated with delayed type hypersensitivity or molecular mimicry and that this is one pathogenic mechanism leading to disease. Serum and mucosal antibodies against cHSP60 among trachoma patients has been shown to be associated with inflammatory and scarring disease [224, 246, 247], while serum antibodies in women have been associated with PID [248–253], tubal factor infertility (TFI), infertility [254], perihepatitis [255] and cervical cancer [249]. In a study of women with TFI compared to women with infertility due to other causes, there was a trend for a higher rate of PBMC proliferative responses when stimulated with cHSP60 compared to EBs for the TFI women, suggesting a possible role in pathogenicity [256]. Similarly, a previous study showed that T lymphocytes from endometrial and fallopian tube tissue from women with PID and TFI responded to cHSP60 stimulation [257]. These findings are supported by studies in the monkey pocket model of salpingitis that showed a delayed type hypersensitivity response to recombinant cHSP60 [258]. A subsequent study in the macaque model lends further support to the role of cHSP60 in delayed type hypersensitivity in fallopian tube pathogenesis where pathology may be mediated by cytotoxic CD8+ T cells [259].

cHSP60 may also play a role in reinfection. Lower levels of IFN-γ produced from cHSP60 stimulation of PBMCs were found to be significantly associated with woman who had *C. trachomatis* reinfection and PID but not women with single infections or infertility due to other causes [260]. In another study, elevated production of IFN-γ from cHSP60 stimulated PBMCs was found to be protective against reinfection [50]. Finally, a recent study found that systemic antibodies to EBs but not cHSP60 were significantly associated with PID recurrence and lower rates of pregnancy over a mean follow-up period of 84 months [253]. Although this is only one study, it suggests that other mediators may be involved in disease or, alternatively, may be markers for infection. Nonetheless, while the source of cHSP60 (e.g. acute or persistent infection) may not be known and there may be no evidence for a productive infection (i.e. culture negative), immune stimulation from cHSP60 – and likely other chlamydial antigens such as PmpD – is thought to cause chronic inflammation and disease [261]. The only caveat is that persistent systemic antibodies may be just a marker for chronic or repeat infection (e.g. cervix or upper genital tract) or for another immune response that is directly involved in pathology. However, in a monkey model of PID, serum antibodies to cHSP60 persisted after treatment and correlated with culture or ligase chain reaction (LCR)-positive tissue [250]. Nonetheless, these data suggest that both an acute and persistent state may be capable of producing virulence factors that mediate inflammation, which can fuel the disease process.

Autoimmunity

There is also some data to suggest that autoimmunity may play a role in disease pathogenesis. cHSP60 has a relatively high sequence homology with the human HSP60 gene. A recent study identified four putative T cell epitopes with 100% homology between the two proteins [262]. In the murine model, a robust T cell proliferative response and high anti-murine HSP60 antibody titers were induced only after immunization with both chlamydial and murine recombinant HSP60 antigens [263]. However, immunization with cHSP60 alone did not have the same effect. There is also homology between the murine heart muscle-specific alpha myosin heavy chain and cHSP60. In murine studies, *C. trachomatis* infection was able to induce antibodies against the myosin protein, while injection of chlamydial HSP60 produced both perivascular inflammation and fibrosis in addition to blockage of heart vessels [264]. The cHSP60 may possess homology to other human proteins that have yet to be identified, which may contribute to urogenital autoimmunity. Nonetheless, it appears that both infection and the host immune response are responsible for pathogenicity and disease outcome.

Host Genetic Susceptibility to Infection and Disease

The above sections have described how infection of epithelial cells by *C. trachomatis* precipitates an innate immune response and inflammation that can resolve or progress if infection is not cleared. A robust adaptive mucosal immune response, including

CD4+ Th1-IFN-γ-producing cells, is important for clearing infection but, with reinfection, may result in host memory T cell defense responses that result in collateral tissue damage. The difficulty in understanding host genetic susceptibility to infection and disease has been well summarized by Taneja and David [265]. Briefly, results are difficult to interpret because of: (1) the genetic variation among individuals even when controlling for ethnic groups; (2) the linkage disequilibrium that exists between HLA class II loci and, thereby, difficulty in linking a single gene to disease, and (3) the limited understanding of autoantigens present at inception of the immune response.

The Role of the Human Leukocyte Antigen
The major histocompatibility complex (MHC) encodes HLA molecules that are highly polymorphic and determine not only the repertoire, but also the specificity of the immune response in humans. HLA molecules are responsible for identifying self from nonself peptides or proteins. Class I antigens present peptides to cytotoxic CD8+ T lymphocytes (CTL) while class II antigens present peptides to CD4+ T cells [266]. Class II haplotypes, which include HLADQ2/DR3, HLA-DQ6/DR2 and HLA-DQ8/DR4, are the most autoimmune-inducing genes and are associated with ~90% of these types of diseases [reviewed in Taneja and David, 265]. CTLs are important in host defense against viruses and intracellular pathogens while CD4+ cells function by inducing antibody and cellular responses to antigens external to the cell.

Reactive arthritis is one of a number of autoimmune diseases that has a multifactorial etiology. This chronic disease is associated with HLA-B27 genetic susceptibility, although the molecular mechanisms remain largely unknown. Environmental factors such as intestinal and urogenital infections with various pathogenic bacteria are proven factors in disease [267]. However, the role of pathogens in spondyloarthritis and other arthropathies is still evolving. *C. trachomatis* is well known as a trigger of reactive arthritis. Indeed, it appears that the HLA B27 B2705* allele is a risk factor for reactive arthritis ascribed to *C. trachomatis*, although it is certainly not present in all cases [268]. An HLA-DRB1*0401-restricted T cell epitope was discovered in the cHSP60, which was recognized by the DR4 clone from a patient with reactive arthritis [269]. A recent study identified two *C. trachomatis* ligands, one of which is a T cell epitope localized to CT610, that appear to engage in molecular mimicry; both peptides were homologous to the HLA-B27 binding motif [270]. These are the first studies to identify specific peptides that may explain the pathogenesis of reactive arthritis in patients with urogenital *C. trachomatis* infections. While there are limited studies of arthritis in animals, a recent study using transgenic mice with HLA class II (DR and DQ) lacking the complete endogenous class II molecules (where expression is similar to that of humans) showed that epistatic interactions between DQ and DR determined progression and severity of inflammatory disease [265].

A limited number of in vitro, animal and human studies have evaluated genetic markers for *C. trachomatis* urogenital infection and the sequelae of PID or tubal factor infertility. In in vitro studies, ~18 strain E MOMP epitopes were found to activate class II HLA-DR1-, 7-, 13-, 17-, DRw52- and DQ3-restricted peripheral blood T cells; two epitopes activated DR4-, 11-, 14- and 18-restricted T cells from men and women with urethral and cervical infections, respectively [271]. Of the class I alleles, 1–5 A2- and B51-restricted epitopes were recognized by CTLs isolated from 10 strain E-infected women with cervicitis compared with 1 of 7 uninfected women [272]. While epitope-specific CTLs were not investigated for association with inflammation, these data suggest a role for class I and II alleles in an adverse host immune response to *C. trachomatis*. In animal models of *C. trachomatis* STDs, 2–5 class I alleles in the pig-tailed macaque correlated with adhesion formation in PID [273]. In mice, immune responses to cHSP60 differed by H-2 haplotype [274]. In humans, DQA*0101 and DQB*0501 were associated with Nairobi sex workers with TFI due to *C. trachomatis*, while DQA*0102 was negatively associated [275]. These latter findings contradict a Finish study where DQA*0102 and DQB*0602 were associated with TFI [276]. Also in Nairobi, DQA1*0401 and DQB1*0402 were associated with high antibody titers to cHSP60, but not with PID [277]. Previously, risk factors for *C. trachomatis* PID in Nairobi included *C. trachomatis* recurrence, serum antibodies against cHSP60, and class I-A31, C2 and C3 [278]. These results represent two populations and limited typing (no DR loci and limited alleles) that are not predictive. One additional study that was conducted in Kenya found that HLA-DR1*1503 and DRB5*0101 appeared to be protective for TFI [279].

There are not many additional recent studies. In one study, incident *C. trachomatis* infection was found to be associated with HLA class II allele DQB1*06 and HLA class I haplotype B*44-Cw*04 [280]. Wang et al. [281] evaluated adolescents at risk for STDs and found that DRB1*03-DQB1*04 and DQB1*06 were significantly associated with recurrent *C. trachomatis* infections measured by the LCR after controlling for the number of sex partners, race, duration of follow-up and other STDs. In addition, the IL-10 promoter G-C-C haplotype (–1,082, –819 and –592) were significantly underrepresented in the population, which correlated with lower IL-10 expression in the cervix. A major limitation of this study was the use of LCR, which was taken off the market due to sensitivity and specificity issues and, thereby, calls into question the diagnostic results. A major drawback of all of these studies, except for the Geisler [221] and Wang et al. [281] studies, is that the diagnosis of *C. trachomatis* infection was made solely on the basis of serological tests, which have limited specificity.

Single Nucleotide Polymorphisms in Immune Response Genes
There is a growing body of knowledge linking the immune response to genetic variation within immune response genes [282]. SNPs can occur in different immune response genes such as TLRs or pathogen recognition receptors that are important in sensing bacteria and triggering host cell signaling after interaction. In a Dutch study, the allele frequency for TLR4 Asp299Gly among TFI patients did not differ from the rest of the population [283]. The findings were similar for a Dutch study of the CD14 functional gene polymorphism –260 C>T [284] and for the IL-1B and IL-1 receptor

agonist among women with TFI [285]. In contrast, an IL-10 promoter polymorphism (1082AA) was found to be associated with TFI [276]. In another study, SNPs in the TLR4, TLR9, CD14 and CARD15/NOD2 were analyzed among Dutch women with laparoscopically confirmed TFI, and a trend in association was found for infertile women with serologic evidence of prior *C. trachomatis* infection who had two or more SNPs [286]. A follow on to the initial study showed that the TLR4 +896 G allele was associated with TFI but not susceptibility to infection [287]. For TLR2, haplotype 1 was associated with protection against infertility among Dutch women with prior infection [288]. In a study of polymorphisms in the mannose-binding lectin among Hungarian women, the codon 54 allele B variant was found to be a risk factor for tubal occlusion compared to controls [289]. Mannose-binding lectin is important in innate immunity in that it can bind to MOMP and block attachment of EBs to the host cell [290]. In studies of the chemokine receptor CCR5 that is involved in T cell function, a CCR5delta32 deletion was noted to be inversely associated with subfertile women [291]. Finally, there are even fewer data among trachoma populations. Atik et al. [292] evaluated SNPs in 36 candidate inflammatory genes and their association with trachomatous trichiasis (defined as more than one lashes touching the eye globe). A significant increase in risk was found with the combination of TNFα (−308G), VDR (intron G), IL4R (50V) and ICAM1 (56M) minor allele. A decrease in risk was associated with the combination TNFα (−308A), LTA (252A), VCAM1 (−1,594C), SCYA 11 (23T) minor allele, and the combination of TNFα (-308A), IL-9 (113M), IL-1B (5′UTR-T) and VCAM1 (−1,594C). While these studies are important, investigations that correlate disease (approved standards techniques for diagnosing endometritis and TFI) with *C. trachomatis* infection (confirmed by reliable nucleic amplification tests or culture) and SNPs where confounding data are controlled for in the analyses will be critical in order to expand and improve our knowledge of host genetic susceptibility to infection and disease.

References

1 World Health Organization: 2011 Initiative for vaccine research. http://www.who.int/vaccine_research/diseases/soa_std/en/index1.html (accessed August 2012).

2 Centers for Disease Control and Prevention: Sexually transmitted disease surveillance, 2009. Atlanta, US Department of Health and Human Services, 2010.

3 Centers for Disease Control and Prevention: *Chlamydia* screening among sexually active young female enrollees of health plans – United States, 2000–2007. MMWR Morb Mortal Wkly Rep 2009;58:362–365.

4 Stamm WE, Jones RB, Batteiger BE: Infectious diseases and their etiologic agents. Section C. Chlamydial Diseases; in Mandell GL, Bennett JE, Dolin R (eds): Principles and Practice of Infectious Diseases. Philadelphia, Churchill Livingston, 2005, pp 2239–2253.

5 Baehr W, Zhang YX, Joseph T, Su H, Nano FE, Everett KD, Caldwell HD: Mapping antigenic domains expressed by *Chlamydia trachomatis* major outer membrane protein genes. Proc Natl Acad Sci USA 1988;85:4000–404.

6 Wang SP, Grayston JT: Three new serovars of *Chlamydia trachomatis*: Da, Ia and L2a. J Infect Dis 1991;163:403–405.

7   Brunham R, Yang C, Maclean I, Kimani J, Maitha G, Plummer F: *Chlamydia trachomatis* from individuals in a sexually transmitted diseases core group exhibit frequent sequence variation in the major outer membrane protein (*omp1*) gene. J Clin Invest 1994; 94:458–463.

8   Dean D: Molecular characterization of new *Chlamydia trachomatis* serological variants from a trachoma endemic region of Africa; in Orfila J, Byrne GI, Chernesky MA, Grayston JT, Jones RB, Ridgway GL, Saikku R, Schachter J, Stamm WE, Stephens RS (eds): Chlamydial Infections. Bologna, Societa Editrice Esculapio, 1994, pp 259–262.

9   Dean D, Patton M, Stephens RS: Direct sequence evaluation of the major outer membrane protein gene variant regions of *Chlamydia trachomatis* subtypes D', I' and L2'. Infect Immun 1991;59:1579–1582.

10 Dean D, Schachter J, Dawson CR, Stephens RS: Comparison of the major outer membrane protein variant sequence regions of B/Ba isolates: a molecular epidemiologic approach to *Chlamydia trachomatis* infections. J Infect Dis 1992;166:383–392.

11 Hayes LJ, Bailey RL, Mabey DC, Clarke IN, Pickett MA, Watt PJ, Ward ME: Genotyping of *Chlamydia trachomatis* from a trachoma-endemic village in the Gambia by a nested polymerase chain reaction: identification of strain variants. J Infect Dis 1992;166: 1173–1177.

12 Lampe MF, Suchland RJ, Stamm WE: Nucleotide sequence of the variable domains within the major outer membrane protein gene from serovariants of *Chlamydia trachomatis*. Infect Immun 1993;61:213–219.

13 Yang CL, Maclean I, Brunham RC: DNA sequence polymorphism of the *Chlamydia trachomatis* omp1 gene. J Infect Dis 1993;168:1225–1230.

14 Hayes LJ, Pecharatana S, Bailey RL, Hampton TJ, Pickett MA, Mabey DC, Watt PJ, Ward ME: Extent and kinetics of genetic change in the *omp1* gene of *Chlamydia trachomatis* in two villages with endemic trachoma. J Infect Dis 1995;172:268–272.

15 Dean D, Oudens E, Bolan G, Padian N, Schachter J: Major outer membrane protein variants of *Chlamydia trachomatis* are associated with severe upper genital tract infections and histopathology in San Francisco. J Infect Dis 1995;172:1013–1022.

16 Frost EH, Deslandes S, Gendron D, Bourgaux-Ramoisy D, Bourgaux P: Variation outside variable segments of the major outer membrane protein distinguishes trachoma from urogenital isolates of the same serovar of *Chlamydia trachomatis*. Genitourin Med 1995;71:18–23.

17 Klint M, Fuxelius HH, Goldkuhl RR, Skarin H, Rutemark C, Andersson SG, Persson K, Herrmann B: High-resolution genotyping of *Chlamydia trachomatis* strains by multilocus sequence analysis. J Clin Microbiol 2007;45:1410–1414.

18 Pannekoek Y, Morelli G, Kusecek B, Morre SA, Ossewaarde JM, Langerak AA, van der Ende A: Multi locus sequence typing of Chlamydiales: clonal groupings within the obligate intracellular bacteria *Chlamydia trachomatis*. BMC Microbiology 2008;8:42.

19 Dean D, Bruno WJ, Wan R, Gomes JP, Devignot S, Mehari T, de Vries HJ, Morre SA, Myers G, Read TD, Spratt BG: Predicting phenotype and emerging strains among *Chlamydia trachomatis* infections. Emerg Infect Dis 2009;15:1385–1394.

20 Fitch WM, Peterson EM, de la Maza LM: Phylogenetic analysis of the outer-membrane-protein genes of *Chlamydia*, and its implication for vaccine development. Mol Biol Evol 1993;10:892–913.

21 Millman KL, Tavare S, Dean D: Recombination in the ompA gene but not the omcB gene of *Chlamydia* contributes to serovar-specific differences in tissue tropism, immune surveillance, and persistence of the organism. J Bacteriol 2001;183:5997–6008.

22 Gomes JP, Bruno WJ, Borrego MJ, Dean D: Recombination in the genome of *Chlamydia trachomatis* involving the polymorphic membrane protein C gene relative to *ompA* and evidence for horizontal gene transfer. J Bacteriol 2004;186:4295–4306.

23 Gomes JP, Bruno WJ, Nunes A, Santos N, Florindo C, Borrego MJ, Dean D: Evolution of *Chlamydia trachomatis* diversity occurs by widespread interstrain recombination involving hotspots. Genome Res 2007;17:50–60.

24 Somboonna N, Wan R, Ojcius DM, Pettengill MA, Joseph SJ, Chang A, Hsu R, Read TD, Dean D: Hypervirulent *Chlamydia trachomatis* clinical strain is a recombinant between lymphogranuloma venereum (L$_2$) and D lineages. mBio 2011;2:e00045–11.

25 Joseph SJ, Didelot X, Gandhi K, Dean D, Read TD: Interplay of recombination and selection in the genomes of *Chlamydia trachomatis*. Biol Direct 2011; 6:28.

26 Joseph SJ, Didelot X, Rothschild J, de Vries HJ, Morre SA, Read TD, Dean D: Population genomics of *Chlamydia trachomatis*: insights on drift, selection, recombination, and population structure. Mol Biol Evol 2012;29:3933–3946.

27 Harris SR, Clarke IN, Seth-Smith HM, Solomon AW, Cutcliffe LT, Marsh P, Skilton RJ, Holland MJ, Mabey D, Peeling RW, Lewis DA, Spratt BG, Unemo M, Persson K, Bjartling C, Brunham R, de Vries HJ, Morre SA, Speksnijder A, Bebear CM, Clerc M, de Barbeyrac B, Parkhill J, Thomson NR: Whole-genome analysis of diverse *Chlamydia trachomatis* strains identifies phylogenetic relationships masked by current clinical typing. Nat Genet 2012;44:413–419.

28 Baud D, Regan L, Greub G: Emerging role of *Chlamydia* and *Chlamydia*-like organisms in adverse pregnancy outcomes. Curr Opin Infect Dis 2008;21: 70–76.

29 Mardh PA: Tubal factor infertility, with special regard to chlamydial salpingitis. Curr Opin Infect Dis 2004;17:49–52.

30 Stamm WE: *Chlamydia trachomatis* infections of the adult; in Holmes K, Sparling P, Stamm WE, Piot P, Wasserheit J, Corey L, Cohen M, Watts H (eds): Sexually Transmitted Diseases. New York, McGraw-Hill, 2008, pp 575–594.

31 Blas MM, Canchihuaman FA, Alva IE, Hawes SE: Pregnancy outcomes in women infected with *Chlamydia trachomatis*: a population-based cohort study in Washington State. Sex Transm Infect 2007;83:314–318.

32 Darville T: *Chlamydia trachomatis* infections in neonates and young children. Semin Pediatr Infect Dis 2005;16:235–244.

33 Anttila T, Saikku P, Koskela P, Bloigu A, Dillner J, Ikaheimo I, Jellum E, Lehtinen M, Lenner P, Hakulinen T, Narvanen A, Pukkala E, Thoresen S, Youngman L, Paavonen J: Serotypes of *Chlamydia trachomatis* and risk for development of cervical squamous cell carcinoma. JAMA 2001;285:47–51.

34 Smith JS, Munoz N, Herrero R, Eluf-Neto J, Ngelangel C, Franceschi S, Bosch FX, Walboomers JM, Peeling RW: Evidence for *Chlamydia trachomatis* as a human papillomavirus cofactor in the etiology of invasive cervical cancer in Brazil and the Philippines. J Infect Dis 2002;185:324–331.

35 Koskela P, Anttila T, Bjorge T, Brunsvig A, Dillner J, Hakama M, Hakulinen T, Jellum E, Lehtinen M, Lenner P, Luostarinen T, Pukkala E, Saikku P, Thoresen S, Youngman L, Paavonen J: *Chlamydia trachomatis* infection as a risk factor for invasive cervical cancer. Int J Cancer 2000;85:35–39.

36 Galvin SR, Cohen MS: The role of sexually transmitted diseases in HIV transmission. Nat Rev Microbiol 2003;2:33–42.

37 Corey L: Synergistic copathogens – HIV-1 and HSV-2. N Engl J Med 2007;356:854–856.

38 McClelland RS, Lavreys L, Katingima C, Overbaugh J, Chohan V, Mandaliya K, Ndinya-Achola J, Baeten JM: Contribution of HIV-1 infection to acquisition of sexually transmitted disease: a 10-year prospective study. J Infect Dis 2005;191:333–338.

39 Cunningham KA, Beagley KW: Male genital tract chlamydial infection: implications for pathology and infertility. Biol Reprod 2008;79:180–189.

40 Gottlieb SL, Berman SM, Low N: Screening and treatment to prevent sequelae in women with *Chlamydia trachomatis* genital infection: how much do we know? J Infect Dis 2010;201(suppl 2):S156–S167.

41 Jones RB, Mammel JB, Shepard MK, Fisher RR: Recovery of *Chlamydia trachomatis* from the endometrium of women at risk for chlamydial infection. Am J Obstet Gynecol 1986;155:35–39.

42 Tu W, Batteiger BE, Wiehe S, Ofner S, Van Der Pol B, Katz BP, Orr DP, Fortenberry JD: Time from first intercourse to first sexually transmitted infection diagnosis among adolescent women. Arch Pediatr Adolesc Med 2009;163:1106–1111.

43 Batteiger BE, Tu W, Ofner S, Van Der Pol B, Stothard DR, Orr DP, Katz BP, Fortenberry JD: Repeated *Chlamydia trachomatis* genital infections in adolescent women. J Infect Dis 2010;201:42–51.

44 Berggren EK, Patchen L: Prevalence of *Chlamydia trachomatis* and *Neisseria gonorrhoeae* and repeat infection among pregnant urban adolescents. Sex Transm Dis 2011;38:172–174.

45 Evans C, Das C, Kinghorn G: A retrospective study of recurrent *chlamydia* infection in men and women: is there a role for targeted screening for those at risk? Int J STD AIDS 2009;20:188–192.

46 van Valkengoed IG, Morre SA, van den Brule AJ, Meijer CJ, Bouter LM, van Eijk JT, Boeke AJ: Follow-up, treatment, and reinfection rates among asymptomatic *Chlamydia trachomatis* cases in general practice. Br J Gen Pract 2002;52:623–627.

47 Hillis SD, Nakashima A, Marchbanks PA, Addiss DG, Davis JP: Risk factors for recurrent *Chlamydia trachomatis* infections in women. Am J Obstet Gynecol 1994;170:801–806.

48 Molano M, Meijer CJ, Weiderpass E, Arslan A, Posso H, Franceschi S, Ronderos M, Munoz N, van den Brule AJ: The natural course of *Chlamydia trachomatis* infection in asymptomatic Colombian women: a 5-year follow-up study. J Infect Dis 2005;191:907–916.

49 Batteiger BE, Lennington W, Newhall WJ, Katz BP, Morrison HT, Jones RB: Correlation of infecting serovar and local inflammation in genital chlamydial infections. J Infect Dis 1989;160:332–336.

50 Brunham RC, Kimani J, Bwayo J, Maitha G, Maclean I, Yang C, Shen C, Roman S, Nagelkerke NJ, Cheang M, Plummer FA: The epidemiology of *Chlamydia trachomatis* within a sexually transmitted diseases core group. J Infect Dis 1996;173:950–956.

51 Morré SA, Rozendaal L, van Valkengoed IG, Boeke AJ, van Voorst Vader PC, Schirm J, de Blok S, van Den Hoek JA, van Doornum GJ, Meijer CJ, van Den Brule AJ: Urogenital *Chlamydia trachomatis* serovars in men and women with a symptomatic or asymptomatic infection: an association with clinical manifestations? J Clin Microbiol 2000;38:2292–2296.

52 Hiltunen-Back E, Haikala O, Kautiainen H, Paavonen J, Reunala T: A nationwide sentinel clinic survey of *Chlamydia trachomatis* infection in Finland. Sex Transm Dis 2001;28:252–258.

53 Rietmeijer CA, Van Bemmelen R, Judson FN, Douglas JM Jr: Incidence and repeat infection rates of *Chlamydia trachomatis* among male and female patients in an STD clinic: implications for screening and rescreening. Sex Transm Dis 2002;29:65–72.

54 Trent M, Chung SE, Forrest L, Ellen JM: Subsequent sexually transmitted infection after outpatient treatment of pelvic inflammatory disease. Arch Pediatr Adolesc Med 2008;162:1022–1025.

55 Niccolai LM, Hochberg AL, Ethier KA, Lewis JB, Ickovics JR: Burden of recurrent *Chlamydia trachomatis* infections in young women: further uncovering the 'hidden epidemic'. Arch Pediatr Adolesc Med 2007;161:246–251.

56 Blythe MJ, Katz BP, Batteiger BE, Ganser JA, Jones RB: Recurrent genitourinary chlamydial infections in sexually active female adolescents. J Pediatr 1992; 121:487–493.

57 Horner P: The case for further treatment studies of uncomplicated genital *Chlamydia trachomatis* infection. Sex Transm Infect 2006;82:340–343.

58 Magbanua JP, Goh BT, Michel CE, Aguirre-Andreasen A, Alexander S, Ushiro-Lumb I, Ison C, Lee H: *Chlamydia trachomatis* variant not detected by plasmid based nucleic acid amplification tests: molecular characterisation and failure of single dose azithromycin. Sex Transm Infect 2007;83:339–343.

59 Gomes JP, Borrego MJ, Atik B, Santo I, Azevedo J, Brito de Sa A, Nogueira P, Dean D: Correlating *Chlamydia trachomatis* infectious load with urogenital ecological success and disease pathogenesis. Microbes Infect 2006;8:16–26.

60 Brunham RC, Pourbohloul B, Mak S, White R, Rekart ML: The unexpected impact of a *Chlamydia trachomatis* infection control program on susceptibility to reinfection. J Infect Dis 2005;192:1836–1844.

61 Atik B, Thanh TT, Luong VQ, Lagree S, Dean D: Impact of annual targeted treatment on infectious trachoma and susceptibility to reinfection. JAMA 2006; 296:1488–1497.

62 Su H, Morrison R, Messer R, Whitmire W, Hughes S, Caldwell HD: The effect of doxycycline treatment on the development of protective immunity in a murine model of chlamydial genital infection. J Infect Dis 1999;180:1252–1258.

63 Carey AJ, Beagley KW: *Chlamydia trachomatis*, a hidden epidemic: effects on female reproduction and options for treatment. Am J Reprod Immunol 2010; 63:576–586.

64 Grayston JT, Wang SP, Yeh LJ, Kuo CC: Importance of reinfection in the pathogenesis of trachoma. Rev Infect Dis 1985;7:717–725.

65 Patton DL, Kuo CC: Histopathology of *Chlamydia trachomatis* salpingitis after primary and repeated reinfections in the monkey subcutaneous pocket model. J Reprod Fertil 1989;85:647–656.

66 Taylor HR, Johnson SL, Prendergast RA, Schachter J, Dawson CR, Silverstein AM: An animal model of trachoma II: the importance of repeated reinfection. Invest Ophthalmol Vis Sci 1982;23:507–515.

67 Hillis SD, Owens LM, Marchbanks PA, Amsterdam LF, Mac Kenzie WR: Recurrent chlamydial infections increase the risks of hospitalization for ectopic pregnancy and pelvic inflammatory disease. Am J Obstet Gynecol 1997;176:103–107.

68 Akande V, Turner C, Horner P, Horne A, Pacey A: Impact of *Chlamydia trachomatis* in the reproductive setting: British Fertility Society Guidelines for practice. Hum Fertil (Camb) 2010;13:115–125.

69 Westrom L, Bengtsson LP, Mardh PA: Incidence, trends, and risks of ectopic pregnancy in a population of women. Br Med J (Clin Res Ed) 1981;282: 15–18.

70 Patton DL, Kuo CC, Wang SP, Halbert SA: Distal tubal obstruction induced by repeated *Chlamydia trachomatis* salpingeal infections in pig-tailed macaques. J Infect Dis 1987;155:1292–1299.

71 Hillis SD, Nakashima AK, Marchbanks PA, Addis DG, Davis J: Risk factors for recurrent *Chlamydia trachomatis* infections in women. Sex Trans Dis 1994;21:S137–S138.

72 Lee V, Tobin JM, Foley E: Relationship of cervical ectopy to *chlamydia* infection in young women. J Fam Plann Reprod Health Care 2006;32:104–106.

73 Carey AJ, Cunningham KA, Hafner LM, Timms P, Beagley KW: Effects of inoculating dose on the kinetics of *Chlamydia muridarum* genital infection in female mice. Immunol Cell Biol 2009;87:337–343.

74 Darville T, Andrews CW Jr, Laffoon KK, Shymasani W, Kishen LR, Rank RG: Mouse strain-dependent variation in the course and outcome of chlamydial genital tract infection is associated with differences in host response. Infect Immun 1997;65:3065–3073.

75 Maxion HK, Liu W, Chang MH, Kelly KA: The infecting dose of *Chlamydia muridarum* modulates the innate immune response and ascending infection. Infect Immun 2004;72:6330–6340.

76 Cotter TW, Miranpuri GS, Ramsey KH, Poulsen CE, Byrne GI: Reactivation of chlamydial genital tract infection in mice. Infect Immun 1997;65:2067–2073.

77 Cocchiaro JL, Valdivia RH: New insights into *Chlamydia* intracellular survival mechanisms. Cell Microbiol 2009;11:1571–1578.

78 Campbell LA, Kuo CC: Interactions of *Chlamydia* with the host cells that mediate attachment and uptake; in Bavoil PM, Wyrick PB (eds): *Chlamydia*: Genomics and Pathogenesis. Norwich, Horizon Bioscience, 2006, pp 505–522.

79 Dautry-Varsat A, Subtil A, Hackstadt T: Recent insights into the mechanisms of *Chlamydia* entry. Cell Microbiol 2005;7:1714–1722.

80 Vretou E, Goswami PC, Bose SK: Adherence of multiple serovars of *Chlamydia trachomatis* to a common receptor on HeLa and McCoy cells is mediated by thermolabile protein(s). J Gen Microbiol 1989; 135:3229–3237.

81 Fudyk T, Olinger L, Stephens RS: Selection of mutant cell lines resistant to infection by *Chlamydia trachomatis* and *Chlamydia pneumoniae*. Infect Immun 2002;70:6444–6447.

82 Jewett TJ, Miller NJ, Dooley CA, Hackstadt T: The conserved Tarp actin binding domain is important for chlamydial invasion. PLoS Pathog 2010;6: e1000997.

83 Lutter EI, Bonner C, Holland MJ, Suchland RJ, Stamm WE, Jewett TJ, McClarty G, Hackstadt T: Phylogenetic analysis of *Chlamydia trachomatis* Tarp and correlation with clinical phenotype. Infect Immun 2010;78:3678–3688.

84 Dean D: Trachoma; in Connor DH, Schwartz DA, Chandler FW (eds): Pathology of Infectious Diseases. Stamford, Appleton and Lange, 1997, pp 498–507.

85 Gerard HC, Stanich JA, Whittum-Hudson JA, Schumacher HR, Carter JD, Hudson AP: Patients with *Chlamydia*-associated arthritis have ocular (trachoma), not genital, serovars of *C. trachomatis* in synovial tissue. Microb Pathog 2010;48:62–68.

86 Whittum-Hudson JA, Gerard HC, Schumacher HR, Hudson AP: Pathogenesis of *Chlamydia*-associated arthritis; in Bavoil PM, Wyrick PB (eds): *Chlamydia*: Genomics and Pathogenesis. Norwich, Horizon Bioscience, 2006, pp 475–504.

87 Rihl M, Kohler L, Klos A, Zeidler H: Persistent infection of *Chlamydia* in reactive arthritis. Ann Rheum Dis 2006;65:281–284.

88 Gerard HC, Whittum-Hudson JA, Carter JD, Hudson AP: The pathogenic role of *Chlamydia* in spondyloarthritis. Curr Opin Rheumatol 2010;22:363–367.

89 Ward ME: Mechanisms of *Chlamydia*-induced diseases; in Stephens RS (ed): *Chlamydia*: Intracellular Biology, Pathogenesis, and Immunity. Washington, ASM Press, 1999, pp 171–221.

90 Norton WL, Lewis D, Ziff M: Light and electron microscopic observations on the synovitis of Reiter's disease. Arthritis Rheum 1966;9:747–757.

91 Ishikawa H, Ohno O, Yamasaki K, Ikuta S, Hirohata K: Arthritis presumably caused by *Chlamydia* in Reiter syndrome: case report with electron microscopic studies. J Bone Joint Surg Am 1986;68:777–779.

92 Schumacher HR Jr, Magge S, Cherian PV, Sleckman J, Rothfuss S, Clayburne G, Sieck M: Light and electron microscopic studies on the synovial membrane in Reiter's syndrome: immunocytochemical identification of chlamydial antigen in patients with early disease. Arthritis Rheum 1988;31:937–946.

93 Gefen O, Balaban NQ: The importance of being persistent: heterogeneity of bacterial populations under antibiotic stress. FEMS Microbiol Rev 2009; 33:704–717.

94 Hannu T, Puolakkainen M, Leirisalo-Repo M: *Chlamydia pneumoniae* as a triggering infection in reactive arthritis. Rheumatology (Oxford) 1999;38: 411–414.

95 Gerard HC, Schumacher HR, El-Gabalawy H, Goldbach-Mansky R, Hudson AP: *Chlamydia pneumoniae* present in the human synovium are viable and metabolically active. Microb Pathog 2000; 29:17–24.

96 Gerard HC, Wang Z, Whittum-Hudson JA, El-Gabalawy H, Goldbach-Mansky R, Bardin T, Schumacher HR, Hudson AP: Cytokine and chemokine mRNA produced in synovial tissue chronically infected with *Chlamydia trachomatis* and *C. pneumoniae*. J Rheumatol 2002;29:1827–1835.

97 Batteiger BE, Fraiz J, Newhall WJ, Katz BP, Jones RB: Association of recurrent chlamydial infection with gonorrhea. J Infect Dis 1989;159:661–669.

98 Kiviat NB, Wolner-Hanssen P, Eschenbach DA, Wasserheit JN, Paavonen JA, Bell TA, Critchlow CW, Stamm WE, Moore DE, Holmes KK: Endometrial histopathology in patients with culture-proved upper genital tract infection and laparoscopically diagnosed acute salpingitis. Am J Surg Pathol 1990;14:167–175.

99 Geisler WM, Whittington WL, Suchland RJ, Stamm WE: Epidemiology of anorectal chlamydial and gonococcal infections among men having sex with men in Seattle: utilizing serovar and auxotype strain typing. Sex Transm Dis 2002;29:189–195.

100 Klint M, Lofdahl M, Ek C, Airell A, Berglund T, Herrmann B: Lymphogranuloma venereum prevalence in Sweden among men who have sex with men and characterization of *Chlamydia trachomatis ompA* genotypes. J Clin Microbiol 2006;44: 4066–4071.

101 Barnes RC, Rompalo AM, Stamm WE: Comparison of *Chlamydia trachomatis* serovars causing rectal and cervical infections. J Infect Dis 1987;156: 953–958.

102 Boisvert JF, Koutsky LA, Suchland RJ, Stamm WE: Clinical features of *Chlamydia trachomatis* rectal infection by serovar among homosexually active men. Sex Transm Dis 1999;26:392–398.

103 Dean D: Chlamydial infections; in Connor DH, Schwartz DA, Chandler FW (eds): Pathology of Infectious Diseases. Stamford, Appleton and Lange, 1997, pp 473–490.

104 Kapoor S: Re-emergence of lymphogranuloma venereum. J Eur Acad Dermatol Venereol 2008;22: 409–416.

105 Stary G, Meyer T, Bangert C, Kohrgruber N, Gmeinhart B, Kirnbauer R, Jantschitsch C, Rieger A, Stary A, Geusau A: New *Chlamydia trachomatis* L2 strains identified in a recent outbreak of lymphogranuloma venereum in Vienna, Austria. Sex Transm Dis 2008;35:377–382.

106 Centers for Disease Control and Prevention: A cluster of lymphogranuloma venereum among men who have sex with men – Netherlands, 2003–2004. MMWR Morb Mortal Wkly Rep 2004;53: 985–988.

107 Martin-Iguacel R, Llibre JM, Nielsen H, Heras E, Matas L, Lugo R, Clotet B, Sirera G: Lymphogranuloma venereum proctocolitis: a silent endemic disease in men who have sex with men in industrialised countries. Eur J Clin Microbiol Infect Dis 2010;29:917–925.

108 Spaargaren J, Fennema HS, Morre SA, de Vries HJ, Coutinho RA: New lymphogranuloma venereum *Chlamydia trachomatis* variant, Amsterdam. Emerg Infect Dis 2005;11:1090–1092.

109 Quinn TC, Taylor HR, Schachter J: Experimental proctitis due to rectal infection with *Chlamydia trachomatis* in nonhuman primates. J Infect Dis 1986; 154:833–841.

110 Dean D: Pathogenesis of chlamydial ocular infections; in Tasman W, Jaeger EA (eds): Duane's Foundations of Clinical Ophthalmology. Philadelphia, Lippincott Williams & Wilkins, 2010, pp 678–702.

111 Dan M, Rotmensch HH, Eylan E, Rubinstein A, Ginsberg R, Liron M: A case of lymphogranuloma venereum of 20 years' duration. Isolation of *Chlamydia trachomatis* from perianal lesions. Br J Vener Dis 1980;56:344–346.

112 Stamm WE: Sexually transmitted diseases; in Holmes K, Sparling P, Stamm WE, Piot P, Wasserheit J, Corey L, Cohen L, Cohen M, Watts H (eds): Sexually Transmitted Diseases. New York, McGraw-Hill, 2008, pp 595–606.

113 El Karoui K, Mechai F, Ribadeau-Dumas F, Viard JP, Lecuit M, de Barbeyrac B, Lortholary O: Reactive arthritis associated with L2b lymphogranuloma venereum proctitis. Sex Transm Infect 2009;85: 180–181.

114 Belland RJ, Zhong G, Crane DD, Hogan D, Sturdevant D, Sharma J, Beatty WL, Caldwell HD: Genomic transcriptional profiling of the developmental cycle of *Chlamydia trachomatis*. Proc Natl Acad Sci USA 2003;100:8478–8483.

115 Tipples G, McClarty G: The obligate intracellular bacterium *Chlamydia trachomatis* is auxotrophic for three of the four ribonucleoside triphosphates. Mol Microbiol 1993;8:1105–1114.

116 Saka HA, Valdivia RH: Acquisition of nutrients by *Chlamydiae*: unique challenges of living in an intracellular compartment. Curr Opin Microbiol 2010; 13:4–10.

117 Grieshaber S, Swanson JA, Hackstadt T: Determination of the physical environment within the *Chlamydia trachomatis* inclusion using ion-selective ratiometric probes. Cell Microbiol 2002;4:273–283.

118 Matsumoto A: Structural characteristics of chlamydial bodies; in Baron AL (ed): Microbiology of *Chlamydia*. Boca Raton, CRC Press, 1988, pp 21–45.

119 Clifton DR, Fields KA, Grieshaber SS, Dooley CA, Fischer ER, Mead DJ, Carabeo RA, Hackstadt T: A chlamydial type III translocated protein is tyrosine-phosphorylated at the site of entry and associated with recruitment of actin. Proc Natl Acad Sci USA 2004;101:10166–10171.

120 Subtil A, Parsot C, Dautry-Varsat A: Secretion of predicted Inc proteins of *Chlamydia pneumoniae* by a heterologous type III machinery. Mol Microbiol 2001;39:792–800.

121 Pennini ME, Perrinet S, Dautry-Varsat A, Subtil A: Histone methylation by NUE, a novel nuclear effector of the intracellular pathogen *Chlamydia trachomatis*. PLoS Pathog 2010;6:e1000995.

122 Subtil A, Delevoye C, Balana ME, Tastevin L, Perrinet S, Dautry-Varsat A: A directed screen for chlamydial proteins secreted by a type III mechanism identifies a translocated protein and numerous other new candidates. Mol Microbiol 2005;56: 1636–1647.

123 Fields KA, Hackstadt T: Evidence for the secretion of *Chlamydia trachomatis* CopN by a type III secretion mechanism. Mol Microbiol 2000;38:1048–1060.

124 Hobolt-Pedersen AS, Christiansen G, Timmerman E, Gevaert K, Birkelund S: Identification of *Chlamydia trachomatis* CT621, a protein delivered through the type III secretion system to the host cell cytoplasm and nucleus. FEMS Immunol Med Microbiol 2009;57:46–58.

125 Muschiol S, Boncompain G, Vromman F, Dehoux P, Normark S, Henriques-Normark B, Subtil A: Identification of a family of effectors secreted by the type III secretion system that are conserved in pathogenic Chlamydiae. Infect Immun 2011;79: 571–580.

126 Chen D, Lei L, Lu C, Flores R, DeLisa MP, Roberts TC, Romesberg FE, Zhong G: Secretion of the chlamydial virulence factor CPAF requires the Sec-dependent pathway. Microbiology 2010;156:3031–3040.

127 Kumar Y, Valdivia RH: Actin and intermediate filaments stabilize the *Chlamydia trachomatis* vacuole by forming dynamic structural scaffolds. Cell Host Microbe 2008;4:159–169.

128 Robertson DK, Gu L, Rowe RK, Beatty WL: Inclusion biogenesis and reactivation of persistent *Chlamydia trachomatis* requires host cell sphingolipid biosynthesis. PLoS Pathog 2009;5:e1000664.

129 Ying S, Pettengill M, Latham ER, Walch A, Ojcius DM, Hacker G: Premature apoptosis of *Chlamydia*-infected cells disrupts chlamydial development. J Infect Dis 2008;198:1536–1544.

130 Pirbhai M, Dong F, Zhong Y, Pan KZ, Zhong G: The secreted protease factor CPAF is responsible for degrading pro-apoptotic BH3-only proteins in *Chlamydia trachomatis*-infected cells. J Biol Chem 2006;281:31495–31501.

131 Buchholz KR, Stephens RS: The extracellular signal-regulated kinase/mitogen-activated protein kinase pathway induces the inflammatory factor interleukin-8 following *Chlamydia trachomatis* infection. Infect Immun 2007;75:5924–5929.

132 Hillis SD, Coles FB, Litchfield B, Black CM, Mojica B, Schmitt K, St. Louis ME: Doxycycline and azithromycin for prevention of chlamydial persistence or recurrence one month after treatment in women: a use-effectiveness study in public health settings. Sex Transm Dis 1998;25:5–11.

133 Somani J, Bhullar VB, Workowski KA, Farshy CE, Black CM: Multiple drug-resistant *Chlamydia trachomatis* associated with clinical treatment failure. J Infect Dis 2000;181:1421–1427.

134 Wang SA, Papp JR, Stamm WE, Peeling RW, Martin DH, Holmes KK: Evaluation of antimicrobial resistance and treatment failures for *Chlamydia trachomatis*: a meeting report. J Infect Dis 2005; 191:917–923.

135 Dreses-Werringloer U, Padubrin I, Jurgens-Saathoff B, Hudson AP, Zeidler H, Kohler L: Persistence of *Chlamydia trachomatis* is induced by ciprofloxacin and ofloxacin in vitro. Antimicrob Agents Chemother 2000;44:3288–3297.

136 Coles AM, Reynolds DJ, Harper A, Devitt A, Pearce JH: Low-nutrient induction of abnormal chlamydial development: a novel component of chlamydial pathogenesis? FEMS Microbiol Lett 1993;106:193–200.

137 Beatty WL, Morrison RP, Byrne GI: Persistent chlamydiae: from cell culture to a paradigm for chlamydial pathogenesis. Microbiol Rev 1994;58:686–699.

138 Caldwell HD, Wood H, Crane D, Bailey R, Jones RB, Mabey D, Maclean I, Mohammed Z, Peeling R, Roshick C, Schachter J, Solomon AW, Stamm WE, Suchland RJ, Taylor L, West SK, Quinn TC, Belland RJ, McClarty G: Polymorphisms in *Chlamydia trachomatis* tryptophan synthase genes differentiate between genital and ocular isolates. J Clin Invest 2003;111:1757–1769.

139 Papp JR, Shewen PE: Localization of chronic *Chlamydia psittaci* infection in the reproductive tract of sheep. J Infect Dis 1996;174:1296–1302.

140 Patton DL, Sweeney YC, Bohannon NJ, Clark AM, Hughes JP, Cappuccio A, Campbell LA, Stamm WE: Effects of doxycycline and antiinflammatory agents on experimentally induced chlamydial upper genital tract infection in female macaques. J Infect Dis 1997;175:648–654.

141 Phillips DM, Burillo CA: Ultrastructure of the murine cervix following infection with *Chlamydia trachomatis*. Tissue Cell 1998;30:446–452.

142 Tau K, Wang H, Suttles J, Campbell W: Persistence of *Chlamydia trachomatis* in the upper genital tracts of experimentally infected mice. Presented at: European Society for *Chlamydia* Research, Stockholm, Uppsala University Centre for STD Research, 2–5 September, 1992

143 Lin JS, Donegan SP, Heeren TC, Greenberg M, Flaherty EE, Haivanis R, Su XH, Dean D, Newhall WJ, Knapp JS, Sarafian SK, Rice RJ, Morse SA, Rice PA: Transmission of *Chlamydia trachomatis* and *Neisseria gonorrhoeae* among men with urethritis and their female sex partners. J Infect Dis 1998;178: 1707–1712.

144 Dean D, Suchland RJ, Stamm WE: Evidence for long-term cervical persistence of *Chlamydia trachomatis* by *omp1* genotyping. J Infect Dis 2000; 182:909–916.

145 Beatty WL, Byrne GI, Morrison RP: Morphologic and antigenic characterization of interferon gamma-mediated persistent *Chlamydia trachomatis* infection in vitro. Proc Natl Acad Sci USA 1993;90: 3998–4002.

146 Beatty WL: Lysosome repair enables host cell survival and bacterial persistence following *Chlamydia trachomatis* infection. Cell Microbiol 2007;9:2141–2152.

147 Ying S, Pettengill M, Ojcius DM, Hacker G: Host-cell survival and death during *Chlamydia* infection. Curr Immunol Rev 2007;3:31–40.

148 Scaffidi P, Misteli T, Bianchi ME: Release of chromatin protein HMGB1 by necrotic cells triggers inflammation. Nature 2002;418:191–195.

149 Bouchard VJ, Rouleau M, Poirier GG: PARP-1, a determinant of cell survival in response to DNA damage. Exp Hematol 2003;31:446–454.

150 Yu H, Schwarzer K, Forster M, Kniemeyer O, Forsbach-Birk V, Straube E, Rodel J: Role of high-mobility group box 1 protein and poly(ADP-ribose) polymerase 1 degradation in *Chlamydia trachomatis*-induced cytopathicity. Infect Immun 2010;78:3288–3297.

151 Zhang YX, Stewart SJ, Caldwell HD: Protective monoclonal antibodies to *Chlamydia trachomatis* serovar- and serogroup-specific major outer membrane protein determinants. Infect Immun 1989;57:636–638.

152 Peeling RW, Brunham RC: Neutralization of *Chlamydia trachomatis*: kinetics and stoichiometry. Infect Immun 1991;59:2624–2630.

153 Su H, Caldwell HD: In vitro neutralization of *Chlamydia trachomatis* by monovalent Fab antibody specific to the major outer membrane protein. Infect Immun 1991;59:2843–2845.

154 Su H, Watkins NG, Zhang YX, Caldwell HD: *Chlamydia trachomatis*-host cell interactions: role of the chlamydial major outer membrane protein as an adhesin. Infect Immun 1990;58:1017–1025.

155 Su H, Morrison RP, Watkins NG, Caldwell HD: Identification and characterization of T helper cell epitopes of the major outer membrane protein of *Chlamydia trachomatis*. J Exp Med 1990;172:203–212.

156 Kim SK, Devine L, Angevine M, DeMars R, Kavathas PB: Direct detection and magnetic isolation of *Chlamydia trachomatis* major outer membrane protein-specific CD8+ CTLs with HLA class I tetramers. J Immunol 2000;165:7285–7292.

157 Ortiz L, Angevine M, Kim S-K, Watkins D, DeMars R: T cell epitopes in variable segments of *Chlamydia trachomatis* major outer membrane protein elicit serovar-specific immune responses in infected humans. Infect Immun 2000;68:1719–1723.

158 Dean D, Millman K: Molecular and mutation trends analyses of *omp1* alleles for serovar E of *Chlamydia trachomatis*: implications for the immunopathogenesis of disease. J Clin Invest 1997;99:475–483.

159 Wang SP, Kuo CC, Barnes RC, Stephens RS, Grayston JT: Immunotyping of *Chlamydia trachomatis* with monoclonal antibodies. J Infect Dis 1985;152:791–800.

160 Hayes LJ, Pickett MA, Conlan JW, Ferris S, Everson JS, Ward ME, Clarke IN: The major outer-membrane proteins of *Chlamydia trachomatis* serovars A and B: intra-serovar amino acid changes do not alter specificities of serovar- and C subspecies-reactive antibody-binding domains. J Gen Microbiol 1990;136:1559–1566.

161 Lampe MF, Kuehl LM, Wong KG, Stamm WE: *Chlamydia trachomatis* major outer membrane protein variants escape neutralization by polyclonal human immune sera; in Orfila J, Byrne GI, Chernesky MA, Grayston JT, Jones RB, Ridgway GL, Saikku P, Schachter J, Stamm WE, Stephens RS (eds): Chlamydial Infections. Bologna, Societa Editrice Esculapio, 1994, pp 91–94.

162 Millman K, Black CM, Johnson RE, Stamm WE, Jones RB, Hook EW, Martin DH, Bolan G, Tavaré S, Dean D: Population-based genetic and evolutionary analysis of *Chlamydia trachomatis* urogenital strain variation in the United States. J Bacteriol 2004;186:2457–2465.

163 Grimwood J, Stephens RS: Computational analysis of the polymorphic membrane protein superfamily of *Chlamydia trachomatis* and *Chlamydia pneumoniae*. Microb Comp Genomics 1999;4:187–201.

164 Lindquist EA, Stephens RS: Transcriptional activity of a sequence variable protein family in *Chlamydia trachomatis*; in Stephens RS, Byrne GI, Christiansen G, Clarke IN, Grayston JT, Rank RG, Ridgway GL, Saikku P, Schachter J, Stamm WE (eds): Chlamydial Infections Proceedings of the Ninth International Symposium on Human Chlamydial Infection. Napa, International *Chlamydia* Symposium, 1998, pp 259–262.

165 Mygind PH, Christiansen G, Roepstorff P, Birkelund S: Membrane proteins PmpG and PmpH are major constituents of *Chlamydia trachomatis* L2 outer membrane complex. FEMS Microbiol Lett 2000;186:163–169.

166 Tanzer RJ, Hatch TP: Characterization of outer membrane proteins in *Chlamydia trachomatis* LGV serovar L2. J Bacteriol 2001;183:2686–2690.

167 Gomes JP, Hsia RC, Mead S, Borrego MJ, Dean D: Immunoreactivity and differential developmental expression of known and putative *Chlamydia trachomatis* membrane proteins for biologically variant serovars representing distinct disease groups. Microbes Infect 2005;7:410–420.

168 Nunes A, Gomes JP, Mead S, Florindo C, Correia H, Borrego MJ, Dean D: Comparative expression profiling of the *Chlamydia trachomatis* pmp gene family for clinical and reference strains. PLoS One 2007;2:e878.

169 Tan C, Hsia RC, Shou H, Haggerty CL, Ness RB, Gaydos CA, Dean D, Scurlock AM, Wilson DP, Bavoil PM: *Chlamydia trachomatis*-infected patients display variable antibody profiles against the nine-member polymorphic membrane protein family. Infect Immun 2009;77:3218–3226.

170 Carlson JH, Porcella SF, McClarty G, Caldwell HD: Comparative genomic analysis of *Chlamydia trachomatis* oculotropic and genitotropic strains. Infect Immun 2005;73:6407–6418.

171 Canaday DH, Wilkinson RJ, Li Q, Harding CV, Silver RF, Boom WH: CD4+ and CD8+ T cells kill intracellular *Mycobacterium tuberculosis* by a perforin and Fas/Fas ligand-independent mechanism. J Immunol 2001;167:2734–2742.

172 Gomes JP, Nunes A, Bruno WJ, Borrego MJ, Florindo C, Dean D: Polymorphisms in the nine polymorphic membrane proteins of *Chlamydia trachomatis* across all serovars: evidence for serovar Da recombination and correlation with tissue tropism. J Bacteriol 2006;188:275–286.

173 Stothard DR, Toth GA, Batteiger BE: Polymorphic membrane protein H has evolved in parallel with the three disease-causing groups of *Chlamydia trachomatis*. Infect Immun 2003;71:1200–1208.

174 Swanson KA, Taylor LD, Frank SD, Sturdevant GL, Fischer ER, Carlson JH, Whitmire WM, Caldwell HD: *Chlamydia trachomatis* polymorphic membrane protein D is an oligomeric autotransporter with a higher-order structure. Infect Immun 2009; 77:508–516.

175 Kiselev AO, Stamm WE, Yates JR, Lampe MF: Expression, processing, and localization of PmpD of *Chlamydia trachomatis* Serovar L2 during the chlamydial developmental cycle. PLoS One 2007;2:e568.

176 Wehrl W, Brinkmann V, Jungblut PR, Meyer TF, Szczepek AJ: From the inside out – processing of the Chlamydial autotransporter PmpD and its role in bacterial adhesion and activation of human host cells. Mol Microbiol 2004;51:319–334.

177 Kawa DE, Stephens RS: Antigenic topology of chlamydial PorB protein and identification of targets for immune neutralization of infectivity. J Immunol 2002;168:5184–5191.

178 Brunelle BW, Sensabaugh GF: The ompA gene in *Chlamydia trachomatis* differs in phylogeny and rate of evolution from other regions of the genome. Infect Immun 2006;74:578–585.

179 Jamison WP, Hackstadt T: Induction of type III secretion by cell-free *Chlamydia trachomatis* elementary bodies. Microb Pathog 2008;45:435–440.

180 Jewett TJ, Fischer ER, Mead DJ, Hackstadt T: Chlamydial TARP is a bacterial nucleator of actin. Proc Natl Acad Sci USA 2006;103:15599–15604.

181 Jewett TJ, Dooley CA, Mead DJ, Hackstadt T: *Chlamydia trachomatis* tarp is phosphorylated by src family tyrosine kinases. Biochem Biophys Res Commun 2008;371:339–344.

182 Clifton DR, Dooley CA, Grieshaber SS, Carabeo RA, Fields KA, Hackstadt T: Tyrosine phosphorylation of the chlamydial effector protein Tarp is species specific and not required for recruitment of actin. Infect Immun 2005;73:3860–3868.

183 Cappello F, Conway de Macario E, Di Felice V, Zummo G, Macario AJ: *Chlamydia trachomatis* infection and anti-Hsp60 immunity: the two sides of the coin. PLoS Pathog 2009;5:e1000552.

184 Read TD, Brunham RC, Shen C, Gill SR, Heidelberg JF, White O, Hickey EK, Peterson J, Utterback T, Berry K, Bass S, Linher K, Weidman J, Khouri H, Craven B, Bowman C, Dodson R, Gwinn M, Nelson W, DeBoy R, Kolonay J, McClarty G, Salzberg SL, Eisen J, Fraser CM: Genome sequences of *Chlamydia trachomatis* MoPn and *Chlamydia pneumoniae* AR39. Nucleic Acids Res 2000;28:1397–1406.

185 Read TD, Myers GS, Brunham RC, Nelson WC, Paulsen IT, Heidelberg J, Holtzapple E, Khouri H, Federova NB, Carty HA, Umayam LA, Haft DH, Peterson J, Beanan MJ, White O, Salzberg SL, Hsia RC, McClarty G, Rank RG, Bavoil PM, Fraser CM: Genome sequence of *Chlamydophila caviae* (*Chlamydia psittaci* GPIC): examining the role of niche-specific genes in the evolution of the Chlamydiaceae. Nucleic Acids Res 2003;31:2134–2147.

186 Thomson NR, Yeats C, Bell K, Holden MT, Bentley SD, Livingstone M, Cerdeno-Tarraga AM, Harris B, Doggett J, Ormond D, Mungall K, Clarke K, Feltwell T, Hance Z, Sanders M, Quail MA, Price C, Barrell BG, Parkhill J, Longbottom D: The *Chlamydophila abortus* genome sequence reveals an array of variable proteins that contribute to interspecies variation. Genome Res 2005;15:629–640.

187 Carlson JH, Hughes S, Hogan D, Cieplak G, Sturdevant DE, McClarty G, Caldwell HD, Belland RJ: Polymorphisms in the *Chlamydia trachomatis* cytotoxin locus associated with ocular and genital isolates. Infect Immun 2004;72:7063–7072.

188 Lyons JM, Ito JI Jr, Pena AS, Morre SA: Differences in growth characteristics and elementary body associated cytotoxicity between *Chlamydia trachomatis* oculogenital serovars D and H and *Chlamydia muridarum*. J Clin Pathol 2005;58:397–401.

189 Thalmann J, Janik K, May M, Sommer K, Ebeling J, Hofmann F, Genth H, Klos A: Actin re-organization induced by *Chlamydia trachomatis* serovar D – evidence for a critical role of the effector protein CT166 targeting Rac. PLoS One 2010;5:e9887.

190 Belland RJ, Scidmore MA, Crane DD, Hogan DM, Whitmire W, McClarty G, Caldwell HD: *Chlamydia trachomatis* cytotoxicity associated with complete and partial cytotoxin genes. Proc Natl Acad Sci USA 2001;98:13984–13989.

191 McClarty G, Caldwell HD, Nelson DE: Chlamydial interferon gamma immune evasion influences infection tropism. Curr Opin Microbiol 2007;10:47–51.

192 Nelson DE, Virok DP, Wood H, Roshick C, Johnson RM, Whitmire WM, Crane DD, Steele-Mortimer O, Kari L, McClarty G, Caldwell HD: Chlamydial IFN-gamma immune evasion is linked to host infection tropism. Proc Natl Acad Sci USA 2005;102:10658–10663.

193 Rottenberg ME, Gigliotti-Rothfuchs A, Wigzell H: The role of IFN-gamma in the outcome of chlamydial infection. Curr Opin Immunol 2002;14: 444–451.

194 Fehlner-Gardiner C, Roshick C, Carlson JH, Hughes S, Belland RJ, Caldwell HD, McClarty G: Molecular basis defining human *Chlamydia trachomatis* tissue tropism: a possible role for tryptophan synthase. J Biol Chem 2002;277:26893–26903.

195 Wood H, Fehlner-Gardner C, Berry J, Fischer E, Graham B, Hackstadt T, Roshick C, McClarty G: Regulation of tryptophan synthase gene expression in *Chlamydia trachomatis*. Mol Microbiol 2003;49: 1347–1359.

196 Akers JC, Tan M: Molecular mechanism of tryptophan-dependent transcriptional regulation in *Chlamydia trachomatis*. J Bacteriol 2006;188:4236–4243.

197 Perry LL, Su H, Feilzer K, Messer R, Hughes S, Whitmire W, Caldwell HD: Differential sensitivity of distinct *Chlamydia trachomatis* isolates to IFN-γ-mediated inhibition. J Immunol 1999;162:3541–3548.

198 Rasmussen SJ, Timms P, Beatty PR, Stephens RS: Cytotoxic-T-lymphocyte-mediated cytolysis of L cells persistently infected with *Chlamydia* spp. Infect Immun 1996;64:1944–1949.

199 Dugan J, Rockey DD, Jones L, Andersen AA: Tetracycline resistance in *Chlamydia suis* mediated by genomic islands inserted into the chlamydial inv-like gene. Antimicrob Agents Chemother 2004;48: 3989–3995.

200 Dugan J, Andersen AA, Rockey DD: Functional characterization of IScs605, an insertion element carried by tetracycline-resistant *Chlamydia suis*. Microbiology 2007;153:71–79.

201 Zhong G, Liu L, Fan T, Fan P, Ji H: Degradation of transcription factor RFX5 during the inhibition of both constitutive and interferon gamma-inducible major histocompatibility complex class I expression in *chlamydia*-infected cells. J Exp Med 2000; 191:1525–1534.

202 Zhong G, Fan T, Liu L: *Chlamydia* inhibits interferon gamma-inducible major histocompatibility complex class II expression by degradation of upstream stimulatory factor 1. J Exp Med 1999;189: 1931–1938.

203 Sharma J, Bosnic AM, Piper JM, Zhong G: Human antibody responses to a *Chlamydia*-secreted protease factor. Infect Immun 2004;72:7164–7171.

204 Sharma J, Dong F, Pirbhai M, Zhong G: Inhibition of proteolytic activity of a chlamydial proteasome/protease-like activity factor by antibodies from humans infected with *Chlamydia trachomatis*. Infect Immun 2005;73:4414–4419.

205 Christian J, Vier J, Paschen SA, Hacker G: Cleavage of the NF-κB family protein p65/RelA by the Chlamydial Protease-like Activity Factor (CPAF) impairs proinflammatory signaling in cells infected with *Chlamydiae*. J Biol Chem 2010;285:41320–41327.

206 Abdul-Sater AA, Said-Sadier N, Ojcius DM, Yilmaz O, Kelly KA: Inflammasomes bridge signaling between pathogen identification and the immune response. Drugs Today (Barc) 2009;45(suppl B):105–112.

207 Abdul-Sater AA, Koo E, Hacker G, Ojcius DM: Inflammasome-dependent caspase-1 activation in cervical epithelial cells stimulates growth of the intracellular pathogen *Chlamydia trachomatis*. J Biol Chem 2009;284:26789–26796.

208 Prantner D, Darville T, Sikes JD, Andrews CW Jr, Brade H, Rank RG, Nagarajan UM: Critical role for interleukin-1β (IL-1β) during *Chlamydia muridarum* genital infection and bacterial replication-independent secretion of IL-1β in mouse macrophages. Infect Immun 2009;77:5334–5346.

209 Hvid M, Baczynska A, Deleuran B, Fedder J, Knudsen HJ, Christiansen G, Birkelund S: Interleukin-1 is the initiator of fallopian tube destruction during *Chlamydia trachomatis* infection. Cell Microbiol 2007;9:2795–2803.

210 Rasmussen SJ, Eckmann L, Quayle AJ, Shen L, Zhang YX, Anderson DJ, Fierer J, Stephens RS, Kagnoff MF: Secretion of proinflammatory cytokines by epithelial cells in response to *Chlamydia* infection suggests a central role for epithelial cells in chlamydial pathogenesis. J Clin Invest 1997;99: 77–87.

211 Abdul-Sater AA, Said-Sadier N, Padilla EV, Ojcius DM: Chlamydial infection of monocytes stimulates IL-1β secretion through activation of the NLRP3 inflammasome. Microbes Infect 2010;12:652–661.

212 Van Voorhis WC, Barrett LK, Sweeney YT, Kuo CC, Patton DL: Analysis of lymphocyte phenotype and cytokine activity in the inflammatory infiltrates of the upper genital tract of female macaques infected with *Chlamydia trachomatis*. J Infect Dis 1996;174:647–650.

213 Scott ME, Ma Y, Farhat S, Shiboski S, Moscicki AB: Covariates of cervical cytokine mRNA expression by real-time PCR in adolescents and young women: effects of *Chlamydia trachomatis* infection, hormonal contraception, and smoking. J Clin Immunol 2006;26:222–232.

214 Wang C, Tang J, Crowley-Nowick PA, Wilson CM, Kaslow RA, Geisler WM: Interleukin (IL)-2 and IL-12 responses to *Chlamydia trachomatis* infection in adolescents. Clin Exp Immunol. 2005;142:548–554.

215 Rank RG, Whittum-Hudson JA: Protective immunity to chlamydial genital infection: evidence from animal studies. J Infect Dis 2010;201(suppl 2):S168–S177.

216 Cain TK, Rank RG: Local Th1-like responses are induced by intravaginal infection of mice with the mouse pneumonitis biovar of *Chlamydia trachomatis*. Infect Immun 1995;63:1784–1789.

217 Perry LL, Feilzer K, Caldwell HD: Immunity to *Chlamydia trachomatis* is mediated by T helper 1 cells through IFN-gamma-dependent and -independent pathways. J Immunol 1997;158:3344–3352.

218 Cotter TW, Ramsey KH, Miranpuri GS, Poulsen CE, Byrne GI: Dissemination of *Chlamydia trachomatis* chronic genital tract infection in gamma interferon gene knockout mice. Infect Immun 1997;65:2145–2152.

219 Morrison SG, Su H, Caldwell HD, Morrison RP: Immunity to murine *Chlamydia trachomatis* genital tract reinfection involves B cells and CD4+ T cells but not CD8+ T cells. Infect Immun 2000;68:6979–6987.

220 Inman RD, Chiu B: Early cytokine profiles in the joint define pathogen clearance and severity of arthritis in *Chlamydia*-induced arthritis in rats. Arthritis Rheum 2006;54:499–507.

221 Geisler WM: Duration of untreated, uncomplicated *Chlamydia trachomatis* genital infection and factors associated with *chlamydia* resolution: a review of human studies. J Infect Dis 2010;201(suppl 2):S104–S113.

222 Brunham RC, Rey-Ladino J: Immunology of *Chlamydia* infection: implications for a *Chlamydia trachomatis* vaccine. Nat Rev Immunol 2005;5:149–161.

223 Agrawal T, Gupta R, Dutta R, Srivastava P, Bhengraj AR, Salhan S, Mittal A: Protective or pathogenic immune response to genital chlamydial infection in women – a possible role of cytokine secretion profile of cervical mucosal cells. Clin Immunol 2009;130:347–354.

224 Skwor TA, Atik B, Kandel RP, Adhikari HK, Sharma B, Dean D: Role of secreted conjunctival mucosal cytokine and chemokine proteins in different stages of trachomatous disease. PLoS Negl Trop Dis 2008;2:e264.

225 Van Voorhis WC, Barrett LK, Sweeney YT, Kuo CC, Patton DL: Repeated *Chlamydia trachomatis* infection of Macaca nemestrina fallopian tubes produces a Th1-like cytokine response associated with fibrosis and scarring. Infect Immun 1997;65:2175–2182.

226 Rank RG, Sanders MM, Patton DL: Increased incidence of oviduct pathology in the guinea pig after repeat vaginal inoculation with the chlamydial agent of guinea pig inclusion conjunctivitis. Sex Transm Dis 1995;22:48–54.

227 Darville T, O'Neill JM, Andrews CW Jr, Nagarajan UM, Stahl L, Ojcius DM: Toll-like receptor-2, but not Toll-like receptor-4, is essential for development of oviduct pathology in chlamydial genital tract infection. J Immunol 2003;171:6187–6197.

228 Patton DL, Taylor HR: The histopathology of experimental trachoma: ultrastructural changes in the conjunctival epithelium. J Infect Dis 1986;153:870–878.

229 Courtright P, Lewallen S, Howe R: Cell-mediated immunity in trachomatous scarring: evidence from a leprosy population. Ophthalmology 1993;100:98–104.

230 Holland MJ, Bailey RL, Hayes LJ, Whittle HC, Mabey DC: Conjunctival scarring in trachoma is associated with depressed cell-mediated immune responses to chlamydial antigens. J Infect Dis 1993;168:1528–1531.

231 Darville T, Hiltke TJ: Pathogenesis of genital tract disease due to *Chlamydia trachomatis*. J Infect Dis 2010;201(suppl 2):S114–S125.

232 Cohen CR, Brunham RC: Pathogenesis of *Chlamydia* induced pelvic inflammatory disease. Sex Transm Infect 1999;75:21–24.

233 Morrison SG, Morrison RP: A predominant role for antibody in acquired immunity to chlamydial genital tract reinfection. J Immunol 2005;175:7536–7542.

234 Grayston JT, Wang SP: The potential for vaccine against infection of the genital tract with *Chlamydia trachomatis*. Sex Transm Dis 1978;5:73–77.

235 Brunham RC, Kuo CC, Cles L, Holmes KK: Correlation of host immune response with quantitative recovery of *Chlamydia trachomatis* from the human endocervix. Infect Immun 1983;39:1491–1494.

236 Cohen CR, Koochesfahani KM, Meier AS, Shen C, Karunakaran K, Ondondo B, Kinyari T, Mugo NR, Nguti R, Brunham RC: Immunoepidemiologic profile of *Chlamydia trachomatis* Infection: importance of heat-shock protein 60 and interferon-γ. J Infect Dis 2005;192:591–599.

237 Arno JN, Ricker VA, Batteiger BE, Katz BP, Caine VA, Jones RB: Interferon-gamma in endocervical secretions of women infected with *Chlamydia trachomatis*. J Infect Dis 1990;162:1385–1389.

238 Grifo JA, Jeremias J, Ledger WJ, Witkin SS: Interferon-gamma in the diagnosis and pathogenesis of pelvic inflammatory disease. Am J Obstet Gynecol 1989;160:26–31.

239 Agrawal T, Vats V, Wallace PK, Salhan S, Mittal A: Cervical cytokine responses in women with primary or recurrent chlamydial infection. J Interferon Cytokine Res 2007;27:221–226.

240 Cotter TW, Meng Q, Shen ZL, Zhang YX, Su H, Caldwell HD: Protective efficacy of major outer membrane protein-specific immunoglobulin A (IgA) and IgG monoclonal antibodies in a murine model of *Chlamydia trachomatis* genital tract infection. Infect Immun 1995;63:4704–4714.

241 Barenfanger J, MacDonald AB: The role of immunoglobulin in the neutralization of trachoma infectivity. J Immunol 1974;113:1607–1617.

242 Lowell GH, Smith LF, Griffiss JM, Brandt BL: IgA-dependent, monocyte-mediated, antibacterial activity. J Exp Med 1980;152:452–457.

243 Yong EC, Klebanoff SJ, Kuo CC: Toxic effect of human polymorphonuclear leukocytes on *Chlamydia trachomatis*. Infect Immun 1982;37:422–426.

244 Murray ES, Charbonnet LT, MacDonald AB: Immunity to chlamydial infections of the eye. I. The role of circulatory and secretory antibodies in resistance to reinfection with guinea pig inclusion conjunctivitis. J Immunol 1973;110:1518–1525.

245 Blake M, Holmes KK, Swanson J: Studies on gonococcus infection. XVII. IgA1-cleaving protease in vaginal washings from women with gonorrhea. J Infect Dis 1979;139:89–92.

246 Hessel T, Dhital SP, Plank R, Dean D: Immune response to chlamydial 60-kilodalton heat shock protein in tears from Nepali trachoma patients. Infect Immun 2001;69:4996–5000.

247 Peeling RW, Bailey RL, Conway DJ, Holland MJ, Campbell AE, Jallow O, Whittle HC, Mabey DC: Antibody response to the 60-kDa chlamydial heat-shock protein is associated with scarring trachoma. J Infect Dis 1998;177:256–259.

248 Peeling RW, Kimani J, Plummer F, Maclean I, Cheang M, Bwayo J, Brunham RC: Antibody to chlamydial hsp60 predicts an increased risk for chlamydial pelvic inflammatory disease. J Infect Dis 1997;175:1153–1158.

249 Paavonen J, Lehtinen M: Interactions between human papillomavirus and other sexually transmitted agents in the etiology of cervical cancer. Curr Opin Infect Dis 1999;12:67–71.

250 Peeling RW, Patton DL, Cosgrove Sweeney YT, Cheang MS, Lichtenwalner AB, Brunham RC, Stamm WE: Antibody response to the chlamydial heat-shock protein 60 in an experimental model of chronic pelvic inflammatory disease in monkeys (*Macaca nemestrina*). J Infect Dis 1999;180:774–779.

251 Eckert LO, Hawes SE, Wolner-Hanssen P, Money DM, Peeling RW, Brunham RC, Stevens CE, Eschenbach DA, Stamm WE: Prevalence and correlates of antibody to chlamydial heat shock protein in women attending sexually transmitted disease clinics and women with confirmed pelvic inflammatory disease. J Infect Dis 1997;175:1453–1458.

252 Ness AR: The response of the rabbit mandibular incisor to experimental shortening and to the prevention of its eruption. Proc R Soc Lond B Biol Sci 1956;146:129–154.

253 Ness RB, Soper DE, Richter HE, Randall H, Peipert JF, Nelson DB, Schubeck D, McNeeley SG, Trout W, Bass DC, Hutchison K, Kip K, Brunham RC: *Chlamydia* antibodies, *chlamydia* heat shock protein, and adverse sequelae after pelvic inflammatory disease: the PID Evaluation and Clinical Health (PEACH) Study. Sex Transm Dis 2008;35:129–135.

254 Ault KA, Statland BD, King MM, Dozier DI, Joachims ML, Gunter J: Antibodies to the chlamydial 60 kilodalton heat shock protein in women with tubal factor infertility. Infect Dis Obstet Gynecol 1998;6:163–167.

255 Money DM, Hawes SE, Eschenbach DA, Peeling RW, Brunham R, Wolner-Hanssen P, Stamm WE: Antibodies to the chlamydial 60 kd heat-shock protein are associated with laparoscopically confirmed perihepatitis. Am J Obstet Gynecol 1997;176:870–877.

256 Kinnunen A, Surcel HM, Halttunen M, Tiitinen A, Morrison RP, Morrison SG, Koskela P, Lehtinen M, Paavonen J: *Chlamydia trachomatis* heat shock protein-60 induced interferon-gamma and interleukin-10 production in infertile women. Clin Exp Immunol 2003;131:299–303.

257 Kinnunen A, Molander P, Laurila A, Rantala I, Morrison R, Lehtinen M, Karttunen R, Tiitinen A, Paavonen J, Surcel HM: *Chlamydia trachomatis* reactive T lymphocytes from upper genital tract tissue specimens. Hum Reprod 2000;15:1484–1489.

258 Patton DL, Sweeney YT, Kuo CC: Demonstration of delayed hypersensitivity in *Chlamydia trachomatis* salpingitis in monkeys: a pathogenic mechanism of tubal damage. J Infect Dis 1994;169:680–683.

259 Lichtenwalner AB, Patton DL, Van Voorhis WC, Sweeney YT, Kuo CC: Heat shock protein 60 is the major antigen which stimulates delayed-type hypersensitivity reaction in the macaque model of *Chlamydia trachomatis* salpingitis. Infect Immun 2004;72:1159–1161.

260 Debattista J, Timms P, Allan J: Reduced levels of gamma-interferon secretion in response to chlamydial 60 kDa heat shock protein amongst women with pelvic inflammatory disease and a history of repeated *Chlamydia trachomatis* infections. Immunol Lett 2002;81:205–210.

261 Kinnunen A, Paavonen J, Surcel HM: Heat shock protein 60 specific T cell response in chlamydial infections. Scand J Immunol 2001;54:76–81.

Dean

262 Campanella C, Marino Gammazza A, Mularoni L, Cappello F, Zummo G, Di Felice V: A comparative analysis of the products of GROEL-1 gene from *Chlamydia trachomatis* serovar D and the HSP60 var1 transcript from Homo sapiens suggests a possible autoimmune response. Int J Immunogenet 2009;36:73–78.

263 Yi Y, Yang X, Brunham RC: Autoimmunity to heat shock protein 60 and antigen-specific production of interleukin-10. Infect Immun 1997;65:1669–1674.

264 Bachmaier K, Neu N, de la Maza LM, Pal S, Hessel A, Penninger JM: *Chlamydia* infections and heart disease linked through antigenic mimicry. Science 1999;283:1335–1339.

265 Taneja V, David CS: Role of HLA class II genes in susceptibility/resistance to inflammatory arthritis: studies with humanized mice. Immunol Rev 2010;233:62–78.

266 Roitt IM: Essential Immunology, ed 8. Oxford, Blackwell Scientific Publications, 1994.

267 Girschick HJ, Guilherme L, Inman RD, Latsch K, Rihl M, Sherer Y, Shoenfeld Y, Zeidler H, Arienti S, Doria A: Bacterial triggers and autoimmune rheumatic diseases. Clin Exp Rheumatol 2008;26:S12–S17.

268 Inman RD: Reactive and enteropathic arthritis; in Klippel JH, Stone JH, Croffford LEJ, White PH (eds): Primer on the Rheumatic Diseases. Atlanta, Arthritis Foundation Press, 2008, pp 217–223.

269 Deane KH, Jecock RM, Pearce JH, Gaston JS: Identification and characterization of a DR4-restricted T cell epitope within *chlamydia* heat shock protein 60. Clin Exp Immunol 1997;109:439–445.

270 Cragnolini JJ, Garcia-Medel N, de Castro JA: Endogenous processing and presentation of T cell epitopes from *Chlamydia trachomatis* with relevance in HLA-B27-associated reactive arthritis. Mol Cell Proteomics 2009;8:1850–1859.

271 Ortiz L, Demick KP, Petersen JW, Polka M, Rudersdorf RA, Van der Pol B, Jones R, Angevine M, DeMars R: *Chlamydia trachomatis* major outer membrane protein (MOMP) epitopes that activate HLA class II-restricted T cells from infected humans. J Immunol 1996;157:4554–4567.

272 Kim SK, Angevine M, Demick K, Ortiz L, Rudersdorf R, Watkins D, DeMars R: Induction of HLA class I-restricted CD8+ CTLs specific for the major outer membrane protein of *Chlamydia trachomatis* in human genital tract infections. J Immunol 1999;162:6855–6866.

273 Lichtenwalner AB, Patton DL, Cosgrove Sweeney YT, Gaur LK, Stamm WE: Evidence of genetic susceptibility to *Chlamydia trachomatis*-induced pelvic inflammatory disease in the pig-tailed macaque. Infect Immun 1997;65:2250–2253.

274 Zhong G, Brunham RC: Antibody responses to the chlamydial heat shock proteins hsp60 and hsp70 are H-2 linked. Infect Immun 1992;60:3143–3149.

275 Cohen CR, Sinei SS, Bukusi EA, Bwayo JJ, Holmes KK, Brunham RC: Human leukocyte antigen class II DQ alleles associated with *Chlamydia trachomatis* tubal infertility. Obstet Gynecol 2000;95:72–77.

276 Kinnunen AH, Surcel HM, Lehtinen M, Karhukorpi J, Tiitinen A, Halttunen M, Bloigu A, Morrison RP, Karttunen R, Paavonen J: HLA DQ alleles and interleukin-10 polymorphism associated with *Chlamydia trachomatis*-related tubal factor infertility: a case-control study. Hum Reprod 2002;17:2073–2078.

277 Gaur LK, Peeling RW, Cheang M, Kimani J, Bwayo J, Plummer F, Brunham RC: Association of *Chlamydia trachomatis* heat-shock protein 60 antibody and HLA class II DQ alleles. J Infect Dis 1999;180:234–237.

278 Kimani J, Maclean IW, Bwayo JJ, MacDonald K, Oyugi J, Maitha GM, Peeling RW, Cheang M, Nagelkerke NJ, Plummer FA, Brunham RC: Risk factors for *Chlamydia trachomatis* pelvic inflammatory disease among sex workers in Nairobi, Kenya. J Infect Dis 1996;173:1437–1444.

279 Cohen CR, Gichui J, Rukaria R, Sinei SS, Gaur LK, Brunham RC: Immunogenetic correlates for *Chlamydia trachomatis*-associated tubal infertility. Obstet Gynecol 2003;101:438–444.

280 Geisler WM, Tang J, Wang C, Wilson CM, Kaslow RA: Epidemiological and genetic correlates of incident *chlamydia trachomatis* infection in North American adolescents. J Infect Dis 2004;190:1723–1729.

281 Wang C, Tang J, Geisler WM, Crowley-Nowick PA, Wilson CM, Kaslow RA: Human leukocyte antigen and cytokine gene variants as predictors of recurrent *Chlamydia trachomatis* infection in high-risk adolescents. J Infect Dis 2005;191:1084–1092.

282 Witkin SS, Linhares I, Giraldo P, Jeremias J, Ledger WJ: Individual immunity and susceptibility to female genital tract infection. Am J Obstet Gynecol 2000;183:252–256.

283 Morré SA, Murillo LS, Bruggeman CA, Pena AS: The role that the functional Asp299Gly polymorphism in the toll-like receptor-4 gene plays in susceptibility to *Chlamydia trachomatis*-associated tubal infertility. J Infect Dis 2003;187:341–343.

284 Ouburg S, Spaargaren J, den Hartog JE, Land JA, Fennema JS, Pleijster J, Pena AS, Morre SA: The CD14 functional gene polymorphism –260 C>T is not involved in either the susceptibility to *Chlamydia trachomatis* infection or the development of tubal pathology. BMC Infect Dis 2005;5:114.

285 Murillo LS, Land JA, Pleijster J, Bruggeman CA, Pena AS, Morre SA: Interleukin-1B (IL-1B) and interleukin-1 receptor antagonist (IL-1RN) gene polymorphisms are not associated with tubal pathology and *Chlamydia trachomatis*-related tubal factor subfertility. Hum Reprod 2003;18:2309–2314.

286 den Hartog JE, Ouburg S, Land JA, Lyons JM, Ito JI, Pena AS, Morre SA: Do host genetic traits in the bacterial sensing system play a role in the development of *Chlamydia trachomatis*-associated tubal pathology in subfertile women? BMC Infect Dis 2006;6:122.

287 den Hartog JE, Lyons JM, Ouburg S, Fennema JSA, de Vries A, Bruggeman CA, Ito JI, Pena AS, Land JA: TLR4 in *Chlamydia trachomatis* infections: knockout mice, STD patients and women with tubal factor subfertility. Drugs Today 2009;45(suppl B):75–82.

288 Karimi O, Ouburg S, de Vries HJC, Pleijster J, Land JA, Morré SA: The role of TLR2 polymorphisms in susceptibility to and severity of *Chlamydia trachomatis* infections. Drugs Today 2009;45:67–74.

289 Sziller I, Babula O, Ujhazy A, Nagy B, Hupuczi P, Papp Z, Linhares IM, Ledger WJ, Witkin SS: *Chlamydia trachomatis* infection, fallopian tube damage and a mannose-binding lectin codon 54 gene polymorphism. Hum Reprod 2007;22:1861–1865.

290 Swanson AF, Ezekowitz RA, Lee A, Kuo CC: Human mannose-binding protein inhibits infection of HeLa cells by *Chlamydia trachomatis*. Infect Immun 1998;66:1607–1612.

291 Barr EL, Ouburg S, Igietseme JU, Morre SA, Okwandu E, Eko FO, Ifere G, Belay T, He Q, Lyn D, Nwankwo G, Lillard J, Black CM, Ananaba GA: Host inflammatory response and development of complications of *Chlamydia trachomatis* genital infection in CCR5-deficient mice and subfertile women with the CCR5delta32 gene deletion. J Microbiol Immunol Infect 2005;38:244–254.

292 Atik B, Skwor TA, Kandel RP, Sharma B, Adhikari HK, Steiner L, Erlich H, Dean D: Identification of novel single nucleotide polymorphisms in inflammatory genes as risk factors associated with trachomatous trichiasis. PLoS One 2008;3:e3600.

Deborah Dean, MD, MPH
Center for Immunobiology and Vaccine Development
Children's Hospital Oakland Research Institute
5700 Martin Luther King Jr. Way, Oakland, CA 94609 (USA)
E-Mail ddean@chori.org

Chapter 3

Black CM (ed): Chlamydial Infection: A Clinical and Public Health Perspective.
Issues Infect Dis. Basel, Karger, 2013, vol 7, pp 61–77 (DOI: 10.1159/000348752)

Chlamydia trachomatis Genome Structure

Timothy E. Putman · Daniel D. Rockey

Department of Biomedical Sciences and the Molecular and Cellular Biology Program,
College of Veterinary Medicine, Oregon State University, Corvallis, Oreg., USA

Abstract

Next generation sequencing approaches have led to completion of several dozen chlamydial genome sequences, most of which are from *Chlamydia trachomatis*. Analysis of these genomes has
shown that chlamydiae, like other obligate intracellular bacteria, have a much reduced genome
structure that implies dependence on the host for much metabolic capability. Certain groups of
genes, including those encoding inclusion membrane proteins and the family of Pmp proteins, have
been significantly expanded against this general reductive evolutionary strategy. Pregenomic and
postgenomic sequence analysis of *C. trachomatis* has led to considerable understanding of nucleotide polymorphisms, insertions and deletions that are associated with certain clinical presentations.
Future research will address chlamydial genome structure in the context of the system in which they
live, and will include data on the host microbiome and host genetic background. We anticipate that
integrating these areas of research will lead to significant progress in our understanding of the nature of chlamydial infection and disease.

There have been many technological revolutions in the study of pathogenic bacteriol-
ogy. These revolutions include the Gram stain and the Petri dish techniques and tools
first described in the 1880s that have routine utility to this day. This era also saw the
first successful efforts to culture bacteria and the association between infection and
disease- critical studies that changed the way we addressed issues of health. Much
more recently, the invention of PCR revolutionized many aspects of science, and allowed specific genetic regions from trace amounts of template to be amplified into a
workable amount of genetic material. PCR and other amplification technologies also
set the table for the latest revolution in biological analysis, which has allowed a completely different set of questions to be asked about infectious disease and almost every
other aspect of biological investigation. This revolution centers on the incredible advances in next generation sequencing, proteomics and computer-aided analysis of
data (i.e. bioinformatics). Advances in these areas are truly spectacular; new tools in
genome sequencing allow vast amounts of DNA to be analyzed both by individuals

and at large sequencing centers. For example, the Department of Energy Joint Genomics Institute, one of several very large-scale sequencing centers worldwide, generated thirty trillion quality bases of nucleotide sequence in the first half of 2012 (updated quarterly statistics available at: http://www.jgi.doe.gov/sequencing/statistics.html). High throughput genome sequencing technologies have undergone significant improvements in the last few years, with genomes such as Chlamydia being sequenceable in just a few days with very little starting material, for a cost of under $100. Advances in proteomics parallel these gains, and the computer-based analysis tools have also kept pace. This has led to an unprecedented availability for researchers and, perhaps soon, the general public of reasonably priced global genetic informatic tools of discovery and diagnosis. These technologies facilitate a truly global analysis of the biology surrounding a host and pathogen, against the background of genetic variability and the myriad unrelated organisms that also exist in this interaction. These advances are touching every aspect of biomedical investigation, from tailoring drug efficacy for individual patient needs (pharmacogenomics), to analysis of microbial participants in complicated disease etiologies. An example of the latter challenge is the use of a systems biology approach to understanding and addressing bacterial vaginosis [1]. As discussed in the previous chapters, chlamydial disease pathogenesis is a function of the intimate interactions between the specific infecting agent and the host immune response. Many of these interactions remain poorly elucidated, and understanding these interactions will be critical to the development of predictive and protective clinical interactions. While the Petri dish and the Gram stain were clearly revolutionary and allowed physicians to rethink the fundamental nature of infectious disease, the current revolution in genomics will facilitate a detailed understanding of disease that until recently could not have been anticipated. The purpose of this chapter will be to address the nature of chlamydial genomics and how the study of genomics has allowed a clearer understanding of the organism and its mechanisms of pathogenesis.

Chlamydia Genome Structure and Evolution

The 'obligate' in obligate intracellular bacteria is a product of requirements by the bacterium to acquire nutrients or anabolic precursors from the host cell. This is commonly reflected in a reduction in both metabolic capability encoded by the parasite, and a concomitant decrease in genome size [2]. This is reflected in the chlamydial genome, where evolution through different levels of animal groups has produced highly syntenous (i.e. similar and similarly ordered) and consistent genomes within the genus *Chlamydia* that are between 1 and 1.2 million base pairs in size [3–8]. This is roughly one fifth to one sixth the size of the *Escherichia coli* and *Pseudomonas aeruginosa* genomes, respectively (web addresses for information on these genomes: v2/pseudomonas.com; genome.wisc.edu/sequencing.htm). This reduction in size reflects a much more limited metabolic diversity and flexibility. A bioinformatic analysis of the chlamydial metabolome indicates that many biosynthetic pathways present in organisms that live outside of cells are absent or severely truncated in the chlamydiae. This includes gene sets associated with amino acid synthesis, nucleotide assembly and other processes involved in free-living growth. In contrast, the chlamydiae have expanded certain lineage-specific gene sets, including those encoding inclusion membrane proteins (Incs) [9], and the polymorphic membrane proteins (Pmps [10]), which, collectively, represent between 6 and 10% of the different genomes. Other chlamydiae-specific proteins that likely function in the intimate interactions between host cell and chlamydiae are the major outer membrane protein (MOMP) [10], the chlamydial proteasome-like activity factor and other proteases [11], the translocated actin-recruiting protein (TARP) [12, 13] and possible mediators of cellular survival and immunity [14–16], some of which are described elsewhere in this chapter or volume.

The unique intracellular niche occupied by chlamydiae has been exploited by *Chlamydia*-like bacteria since before vertebrates evolved. Analysis of genome sequences from parachlamydiae and protochlamydiae demonstrate that this lineage of bacteria has continued to manicure and reduce its genomic capability as the chlamydiae have become more completely dependent on the host, and have discarded genes that become 'extra baggage' in this environment [2]. This model of chlamydial evolution is consistent with genomic structures of many different bacteria, both intracellular and extracellular, that have evolved to an intimate and dependent interaction with a particular host. For example, the obligately intracellular rickettsiae have genome sizes similar to chlamydiae [17, 18], while *Treponema pallidum* (1.1 megabase genome) [19] and *Mycoplasma* spp. (0.6–1.3 megabase genomes) [20], each of which are fastidious extracellular bacteria that are intimately intertwined with host mucosal environments, have similarly-sized or smaller genomes.

Many chlamydiae also carry a remarkable small plasmid that has recently been correlated with virulence [21, 22]. The presence of the plasmid is noteworthy for several reasons. This highly conserved genetic element in many ways is quite different to plasmids in other systems, where these mosaic and ever changing genetic elements are used to shuffle genetic capability among strains and species, variably integrating into the chromosome or being maintained extrachromosomally, adding overall variability to the genetic capability of a species [reviewed in 23]. In *Chlamydia trachomatis*, however, the plasmid is another example of consistency among genomes, with differences in plasmid presence and structure being the rare exception. The plasmid encodes eight open reading frames, at least one of which is important to virulence [24].

Variation in chlamydial plasmid structure has recently led to problems in diagnosis of chlamydial infections, as the target of a routinely used commercial amplification-based assay was specific to a deleted region of the plasmid, leading to expansion of a strain in patients that were falsely identified as uninfected [25].

Some of the flow of evolution can be observed in the analysis of genome structure of organisms related to the chlamydial pathogens of humans; this includes the members of the genera *Parachlamydia*, *Protochlamydia*, *Simkania* and *Waddlia* (fig. 1).

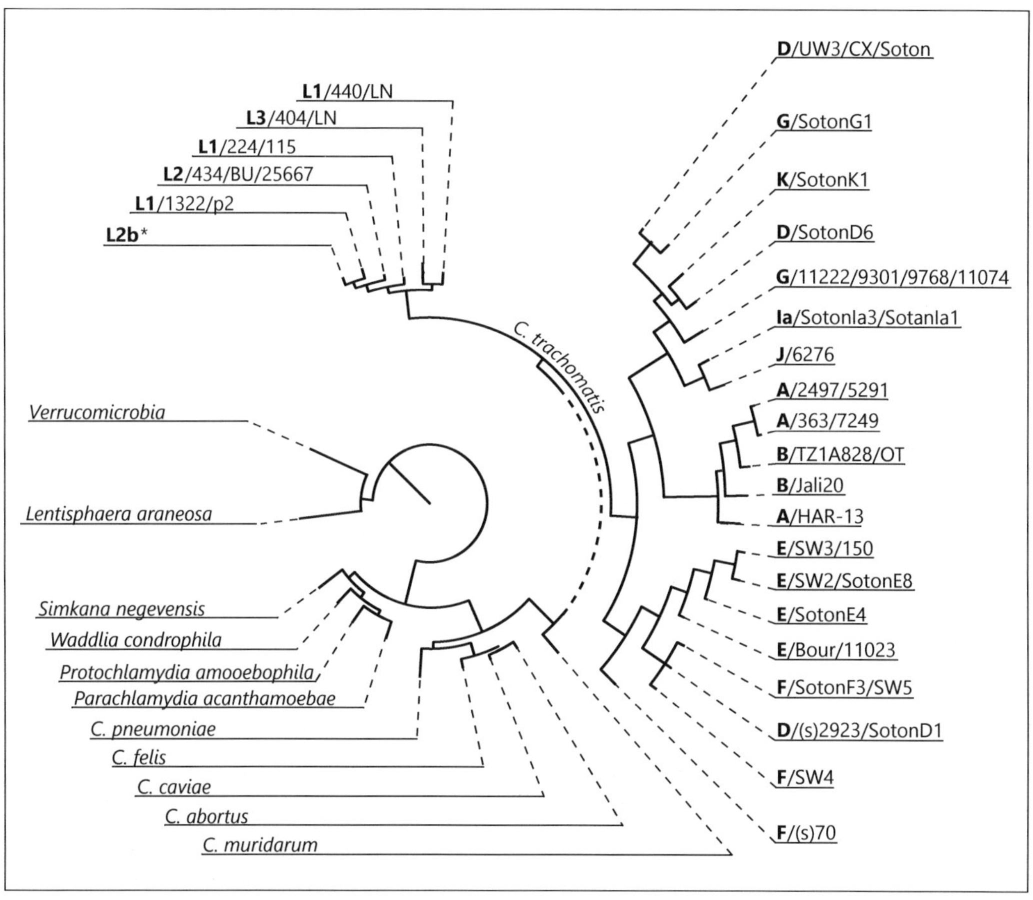

Fig. 1. Phylogeny of *Chlamydia* and closely related species with strain resolution for *C. trachomatis* [data from references 26 and 57].

Most of these related organisms also encode certain proteins that are considered essential to the chlamydial lineage. A highly conserved type III secretion machine is encoded by each of these groups, and it is postulated that this important and widely distributed tool for interacting directly with host cells might have evolved originally in an organism on this lineage. While different members of the lineage will lack one or another of the proteins described in the above paragraphs, evolution or acquisition of genes encoding these proteins appear to be among the most important players in the exploitation of the chlamydial intracellular niche by the evolving *Chlamydia*-like bacteria [26].

The considerable synteny of the chlamydial genome makes it both straightforward and challenging to identify regions of sequence variability that are important to differences in pathogenicity. A comparison of each of the *C. trachomatis* genomes shown in figure 1 demonstrates that there are very few loci in the genome that are highly

Table 1. Identification of the most highly variable *C. trachomatis* open reading frames across all sequenced genomes

Designation	Protein	DNA % diff.	AA % diff.	Gene name	Function	Reference
CT046	NP_219549.1	2.44	1.34	*hctB*	histone-like protein 2	[60]
CT049	NP_219552.1	6.56	10.17		hypothetical protein	[61]
CT050	NP_219553.1	6.39	18.73		hypothetical protein	
CT051	NP_219554.1	5.21	10.38		hypothetical protein	
CT144	NP_219647.1	2.57	3.99		hypothetical protein	[62]
CT166*	NP_219669.1	19.73	15.06		glucosyltransferase	[63]
CT173*	NP_219677.1	20.02	21.25		hypothetical protein	
CT413	NP_219923.1	6.4	1.45	*pmpB*	polymorphic outer membrane protein	[64]
CT414	NP_219924.1	5.3	1.91	*pmpC*	polymorphic outer membrane protein	[64]
CT442	NP_219954.1	2.14	4.15		hypothetical protein	[65]
CT456	NP_219969.1	3.08	8.38		hypothetical protein	[62]
CT619	NP_220136.1	3.24	5.22		hypothetical protein	[62]
CT649	NP_220167.1	2.18	3	*ygfA*	formyltetrahydrofolate synthetase	
CT651	NP_220169.1	2.21	2.37		hypothetical protein	
CT652	NP_220170.1	2.37	1.83	*recD_2*	exodeoxyribonuclease V alpha chain	
CT675	NP_220194.1	2.09	1.04	*karG*	ATP guanido phosphotransferase	[62]
CT677	NP_220196.1	3.29	1.14	*frr*	ribosomal recycling/release factor	
CT679	NP_220198.1	3.54	2.59	*tsf*	elongation factor	[62]
CT680	NP_220199.1	4.03	3.59	*rpsB*	30S-S2 ribosomal	
CT681	NP_220200.1	5.98	8.56	*ompA*	major outer membrane protein	
CT748	NP_220267.1	2.04	0.6	*mfd*	transcription-repair coupling factor	
CT852	NP_220374.1	2.43	3.23	*yhgN*	YhgN family-integral membrane protein	[62]
CT869	NP_220391.1	3.97	2.37	*pmpE*	polymorphic outer membrane protein	[64]
CT870	NP_220392.1	5.73	4.23	*pmpF*	polymorphic outer membrane protein	[64]
CT872	NP_220394.1	2.55	2.05	*pmpH*	polymorphic outer membrane protein	[64]
CT873	NP_220395.1	3.09	2.24		hypothetical protein	

* Indicates genes that are not represented in LGV strains.

variable across the species (table 1), and there are no examples within *C. trachomatis* of genuine genomic islands seen in many other pathogenic species. This is in contrast to many pathogenic species that cause diseases of humans or animals, but is consistent with highly evolved intracellular pathogens. Variability in *E. coli*, for example, is spread across the genome and there are large genomic islands (i.e. pathogenicity islands) that clearly define differences in tropism, disease capacity, or antibiotic resistance among strains [27]. There is a single genomic island found in *Chlamydia* spp. – the 'tet(C) island' of *C. suis* [28], a classic antibiotic resistance element that was acquired from unrelated bacteria [29]. This island allows these organisms to survive in an animal husbandry environment that has historically included subtherapeutic administration of tetracycline as a growth promoter. These strains are found worldwide [30] and the resistance allele can be transferred to *C. trachomatis* in the laboratory [31], demonstrating that human pathogenic chlamydiae can become resistant to antibiotics that are commonly used to treat such infections. Outside of this genomic island, *Chlamydia* spp. tend to vary by differently inactivating, deleting duplicating or modifying individual genes from within the lineage. The following sections will describe individual coding sequences and proteins that vary among chlamydial strains, with a goal of addressing how these proteins might affect differences in pathogenesis.

Variation in Genome Structure within *C. trachomatis*

ompA (CT681)

Identification of genomic regions of variability within the *C. trachomatis* genome began before genome sequences in this system were possible. Initial examples of genomic diversity centered on variation in *ompA*, the gene encoding MOMP, which is the major serovariant antigen in *C. trachomatis* and other chlamydiae [10]. Serotypic differences among different chlamydiae were characterized with antibodies to MOMP, and these differences were associated with differences in disease spectrum among strains. Strains of serovars A, B and C were associated primarily with Trachoma, serovars D-K with classical urogenital chlamydial disease, and serovars L1, L2 and L3 associated with lymphogranuloma venereum (LGV), a more aggressive and invasive condition. Sequence analysis of MOMP identified four major hypervariable regions, which represent the primary regions of the protein that are exposed to the surface [32]. These primary sequencing experiments also demonstrated that recombination occurred among chlamydial strains, leading to MOMP proteins that are mosaics of different serovars [33].

The Chlamydial Plasticity Zone (CT152–176)

The first four chlamydial genome sequences to be completed included *C. trachomatis* serovar D, *C. pneumoniae* AR39 and CWL029, and *C. muridarum* Nigg. A comparative genomics analysis by one of the groups conducting this sequencing included a discussion of a 20–50 kB region of the genome that varies considerably among these four strains, against the described background of considerable sequence similarity and synteny [6]. Continued exploration of chlamydial genome sequences demonstrates that this region is variable across the genus *Chlamydia* [6]. This region of the chromosome contains several candidate virulence factors that may play a role in why these pathogens target different species (i.e. mouse or human) and/or different tissues within species (i.e. lung, genital tract or eye). A walk through the plasticity zone in *C. trachomatis* and *C. muridarum* highlights the possible role of some of these differences.

Tryptophan Synthesis

The amino acid tryptophan has long held a curious place in chlamydial biology. It has been known that starving cells of tryptophan in vitro, or of one of several other amino acids, leads to interruption of the classical developmental cycle and the formation of division-incompetent reticulate bodies that do not mature to elementary bodies [34].

These aberrant forms likely have a unique place in disease pathogenesis associated with chlamydial infection. The role of tryptophan in *C. trachomatis*-host interactions followed the determination that, in human cells, exogenous interferon gamma upregulates the production of indoleamine deoxygenase, a protein that depletes intracellular tryptophan abundance [35]. Thus, the cell is working to reduce the ability of the intracellular pathogen to grow, by removing this important building block from the nutrient pool.

This story becomes even more interesting when variation in tryptophan biosynthetic machinery is compared among the different chlamydial strains. The genes *trpA* (CT171) and *trpB* (CT 170) are present in the plasticity zone of *C. trachomatis* strains, while these genes (and any other fragment of the Trp biosynthetic machinery) are absent in the closely related *C. muridarum* [5]. Expression of intact chlamydial *trp*A/B in *E. coli* demonstrated that they were functional, and that they led to the ability of strains to metabolize tryptophan from indole. Analysis of a large collection of strains in the University of Washington Chlamydia Repository demonstrated that *trp*A/B in ocular strains of *C. trachomatis* are inactivated by deletions introducing frameshifts, while these genes are intact in strains and serovars that grow in the genital tract [36]. This distinction is amplified when serovar B is considered. Strains of this serovar can be divided into those that cause blinding trachoma and those that cause classic urogenital disease. In each strain, the genotype at *trp*A/B is consistent with the target tissue of the infection. There is considerable variation in the *trp* loci among the different chlamydial species, likely reflecting their need to differently exploit the host-based nutritional condition and stresses in each of their target hosts [6].

Differences in the Trp operon among different *C. trachomatis* strains represent a fascinating example of how genome structure allows these organisms to exploit a particular host niche. Why would a pathogen of the genital tract be selected for an ability to metabolize indole to tryptophan, while a strain that grows in the conjunctivae specifically lacks this ability? The answer could come from the nature of the microbiota in each environment. The lower genital tract is colonized by a large variety of organisms that likely can provide some level of indole to the community. This is not the case in the conjunctivae, where the abundance and diversity of the microbiota is much lower. Therefore, chlamydiae infecting the genital tract have the opportunity to exploit a nutritional source that allows them to grow in a hostile environment that may be replete with IFN-γ-secreting T cells, which are working to starve the intracellular bacteria for tryptophan. While the T cells are likely present as well in the conjunctivae, the source of indole might be lacking, leading to a reduced need for the ability to metabolize this product.

C. trachomatis and *C. muridarum* also encode partial or complete fragments, respectively, of a large protein sharing identity with cellular cytotoxins from other species [37, 38]. Treatment of host cells with homologous toxins from other species (e.g. *Clostridium difficile* and *E. coli*) leads to cytoskeletal rearrangement resulting from disruption of host cell GTPase activity. Within the chlamydiae, the number and structure of these toxins varies among and within species. For example, *C. muridarum* encodes three copies of this toxin, while different *C. trachomatis* strains carry different fragments or frameshifted regions of the toxin open reading frame. *C. trachomatis* serovars L1–L3 encode very short fragments of the toxin, and almost certainly express no toxin activity; one exception being a recombinant L2 strain discussed later in this chapter. Hypotheses surrounding the role of these toxins in the differential tissue tropism and pathogenesis of different *C. trachomatis* strains have been challenging.

Other plasticity zone genes vary among strains (e.g. CT149–151) [39], but it is not clear how the presence or absence of these coding sequences participates in the different tropisms and clinical presentations observed within *C. trachomatis*. The plasticity zone is the one region of the chlamydial chromosome in which reductive evolution is still in progress, and changes in this region have likely been selected for optimal growth in the different environments occupied by these otherwise closely related strains and species.

Pmps, Incs and TARP
There are several other genes that vary in structure across the *C. trachomatis* genome, including some that might have a role in host and tissue specificity. The two large families of genes mentioned earlier in the review – the Pmps and the Incs – are present across the chlamydial lineage, and vary significantly across the species. For example, chlamydial Pmps, which are members of the autotransporter (i.e. type V) family of secreted proteins, are scattered across all *Chlamydia* spp. genomes. The effector domains of these proteins are secreted out of the chlamydial developmental forms and *C. trachomatis* has over 10 different *pmp* or *pmp*-like genes, while *C. pneumoniae* has expanded this family to over 20. The encoded proteins have a variety of functions in chlamydial biology, and there are differences in the number of Pmps between species and differences in the sequence of Pmps within species. This pattern is also found in the chlamydial Inc proteins. The number and structure of Incs vary both across and within species, with significant differences observed among the different human pathogenic species. Although there are excellent examples where gene function has been elucidated for Incs and Pmps, the study of these proteins remains in its infancy. It is possible that differences in abundance and sequence of Pmps and Incs have a significant role in the interactions of the different chlamydiae with different hosts and host cells.

The chlamydial TARP (CT 456) functions in early interactions between chlamydiae and the host cell, facilitating primary uptake through major rearrangements of actin in the host cell [12, 13]. TARP from each species contains actin-binding domains and a proline-rich domain; TARP from strains within *C. trachomatis* also have a tyrosine-rich phosphorylation domain. It is proposed that the proline-rich domain facilitates TARP-TARP interactions which focus the actin nucleation events, facilitating uptake. It is not clear how that phosphorylation domain participates in this process, as it is absent from the *C. trachomatis* strains examined to date. Structural differences are present in TARP both within and between species [40], and differences in TARP structure correlate with the differences in invasive characteristics of *C. trachomatis* [41].

Smaller Scale Genetic Variation and Disease Pathogenesis

We have discussed the overall synteny and conservation of genome structure in *C. trachomatis*, and how it is likely that genetic differences such as *trpA/B* structure likely participate in the variety of diseases that are caused by these pathogens. There is also evidence that *C. trachomatis* genetic variation within an individual patient might lead to variation in different disease outcomes in that patient, or perhaps in patient partners following transmission of the pathogen. Data exists supporting a model that single nucleotide polymorphisms exist in strains from clinical samples that may significantly affect the biology of the pathogen in vivo. An example of this was first uncovered in patients persistently infected with a serovar I strain [42]. These individuals were positive for the same serovar of *C. trachomatis* for many months or even years, and a subsequent study showed that the infecting chlamydiae expressed a variable phenotype in culture over the course of their infections. Isolated and cloned *C. trachomatis* from these individuals expressed either a fusogenic or nonfusogenic inclusion phenotype, which is correlated with the presence or absence of an inclusion membrane protein, IncA (CT 119) [43, 44]. A retrospective analysis of patients infected with IncA-negative (i.e. nonfusogenic) strains demonstrated that this genotype was associated with lower infectious organisms and clinical symptoms in the patient [45]. Subsequent work demonstrated that individual strains infecting patients can be a mixture of IncA-negative and IncA-positive clones, and that genomic decay likely leads to switching of this phenotype in vivo [44].

A second gene that varied in the patients infected with a mixture of IncA-postive and IncA-negative, highly related strains was CT135, a hypothetical gene that was variably intact or interrupted in different infecting strains. While the function of CT135 remains unclear, its role as a virulence factor was demonstrated by Sturdevant et al., [46] who showed that laboratory strains of *C. trachomatis* contain subpopulations that have deletions in this open reading frame, and that these deletions lead to differences in the ability of the pathogen to colonize the upper genital tract in a murine model system. These studies support a hypothesis that chlamydial strains in patients are likely pools of strains that vary at different positions in the genome, and that these differences affect tissue tropism and other aspects of disease. Other phenotypes might also vary in vivo [47] and there is good evidence that many routinely used *C. trachomatis* strains exist as pools of organisms that differ slightly at many positions in the genome. This is also supported by primate studies that show subtle genetic differences can lead to significant differences in pathology in a primate model of Trachoma [48]. The study of additional areas of genomic variation continues in many laboratories [39, 48, 49], and it is likely that elucidation of the functions associated with such differences will greatly enhance our ability to understand differences in pathogenesis among strains.

Efforts to Develop Molecular Typing Strategies

Historically, *Chlamydia* infections of many species were diagnosed through the use of specific antibodies to either the group-specific lipopolysaccharide molecule, or the serovariant major outer membrane protein. Highly specific antibodies were generated for these studies, and such analyses remain useful in some diagnostic and research settings. NAATS-based approaches for diagnosis of infection followed the advent of PCR, leading to urine-based diagnostics that are minimally invasive. While there have been examples of problems with these assays, in general they are excellent tools for diagnostic analysis and epidemiology. However, these analyses remain limited to plus/minus-type infection studies, where very little of the nature of the infecting organism can be assessed. As the body of knowledge of individual *Chlamydia* genome sequences has expanded, different strategies have emerged to facilitate both identification of *Chlamydia*-infected individuals and to work toward mechanisms to correlate individual chlamydial genotype with a specific pathologic process. The following paragraphs will address these new developments.

Multilocus Sequence Typing

The multilocus sequence typing (MLST) approach works to examines genetic polymorphisms in a relatively limited number of loci, with a goal of evaluating as many group-specific differences as possible. A variety of multilocus sequence typing profiles for chlamydiae have been developed by different laboratories, each based on a set of between 5 and 7 different genetic sequences in the *Chlamydia* genome [50–53] (table 2). A different set of assays are based on tandem repeat sequences (e.g. multilocus variable number tandem repeat analysis) [54, 55] which can also be used as epidemiologic markers for different strains. While these strategies are clearly useful in the understanding of epidemiologic patterns in chlamydial infections, their utility in understanding differences in disease progression in patients remains to be elucidated. It is likely that continued advances in next-gen sequencing technologies will significantly affect our ability to conduct these analyses on a larger number of loci, leading to clearer definitions of strains for epidemiologic purposes.

Strain Evolution and Emergence

As mentioned earlier, original understandings of *C. trachomatis* strain variation was limited to the analysis of the different serotypes, which led to ~18 canonical serovars. As sequencing technologies improved, variation at many loci (e.g. *trp*, plasticity zone,

Table 2. Summary of contemporary sequence typing systems for genotyping different *C. trachomatis* strains

Group [reference]	Method	Loci	Strains n	Sequence types, n	Description
Klint et al. [50]	MLST	CT046, CT058, CT144, CT172, CT682	47	32	5 hypervariable regions including 3 hypothetical genes
Pannekoek et al. [53]	MLST	CT587, CT855, CT0003, CT498, CT742, CT371, CT198	26	15	7 housekeeping genes
Dean et al. [66]	MLST	CT432, CT376, CT245, CT653, CT332, CT781, CT209	87	44	7 housekeeping genes
Pannekoek et al. [53]	*omp1*-VNTR	CT642-CT643 (intergenic), CT259-CT260 (intergenic), CT172, CT681	93	87	4 variable number tandem repeat loci including intergenic regions and *ompA*
Pedersen et al. [54]	MLVA-5	CT046, CT456, CT632-CT633 (intergenic), CT868, CT872	43	15	5 variable number tandem repeat loci including intergenic regions

Indicated loci numbers are based on the annotations from the *C. trachomatis* D/UW3 genome sequence.

the Pmps) led to understanding that variation clearly extended beyond serotype, and that many individual genetic variations might correlate with differences in disease and tissue tropism. Whole genome sequencing has greatly expanded our understanding of this issue. Sequence analysis has led to the identification of chlamydial genomes that are clear mosaics of different canonical serotypes, with variation not being observed at loci that have been previously associated with differences in pathogenesis or serovariation. The first of these were uncovered by Jeffrey et al. [49], who determined that an IncA-negative variant strain (Ds/2923) contains a D *ompA* gene within a genetic background more closely related to E and F strains (fig. 1). This manuscript also shows evidence of recombination within an F variant strain, in regions of the chromosome that are different to those shown in Ds/2923. Work by Dean and colleagues also addresses this issue – these individuals have identified a unique recombinant strain that is a hybrid between strains of serovars D and L2, resulting in a strain with unusual growth characteristics and an apparently 'hypervirulent' phenotype. Notably, this recombinant L2 strain has an intact toxin gene (CT166; table 1), which is absent in other LGV strains as discussed earlier in this chapter, and is associated with severe hemorrhagic proctitis in vivo, and an in vitro cytotoxicity not seen in other L2 strains [56].

Examples of apparently random recombination across the genome of clinical chlamydial isolates was confirmed and greatly expanded by Harris et al. [57], who added a large and significant list of sequenced strains to the genome database. These studies support a model in which recombination is widespread in *C. trachomatis* strains, likely occurring in patients, and perhaps resulting in phenotypic switching among these generally closely related strains. Issues that remain in this area include the mechanism of DNA exchange by chlamydiae, the actual role of this recombination in chlamydial biology and disease, and the possibility that recombination hotspots are used during chlamydial lateral gene transfer [58].

While much of the discussion here centers on gene-level or genome-level changes that affect pathogenesis of individual chlamydial strains, the role of small variations in genome structure, or simply the emergence of otherwise highly related strains in a susceptible host population, remains important in this system. For example, a unique LGV isolate (L2b) has been found recently in Europe and Canada [59]. The L2b *ompA* sequence of the L2b strains was identical to that found in strains archived in San Francisco in the 1980's, indicating that this strain lineage has been expanding into susceptible populations for at least 25 years. Harris and colleagues sequenced 12 contemporary isolates of the L2B lineage when they conducted their large-scale genome sequencing study [57], and showed that there was a maximum of 19 sequence differences between the members of that lineage. The precise genetic or social changes that led to the expansion of this clone remain unclear. However, there are differences in the *ompA* gene that likely reflect differences in MOMP antigenicity. Also, as discussed above, previous work in a primate system suggests that such differences can be critical to immune avoidance *C. trachomatis* infections [48]. The L2b story likely represents a very good model of how *C. trachomatis* strains ebb and flow among patient populations, and the associated slow sequence changes that occur is complemented by recombination events between strains in multiply-infected individuals, leading to perhaps a larger reshuffling of genetic and phenotypic differences among *C. trachomatis* in human populations.

Sequencing of host genes that participate in chlamydial disease pathogenesis plus the radical technological advances in bioinformatic analysis has allowed a novel field to develop, the field of 'public health genomics'. The driving concept in this area is the integration of individual genome sequences and human genetic polymorphisms into the therapeutic options that might be most applicable in a single infected patient. This approach is a developing area in chlamydial biology, but researchers still have a long way to go. Several different laboratories have worked in this area, with a goal of identifying host genetic variants that are associated with either enhanced pathology or reduced disease in the patient population (table 3). There is a useful presentation of many of these genes in the chapter by Dean in this volume, and we will not repeat these discussions here. Much of these data can be compared to experiments with murine model systems, either through analysis of knockout mice or analysis of microarray data. These are particularly challenging experiments, as the readout needs to be clearly defined and complicating comorbidity determinants have to be carefully addressed. The accumulating data suggests that variation in several different genes encoding proteins participating in the immune response are associated with disease severity, including genes encoding HLA molecules, cytokines and Toll-like receptors. As technologies for accumulating and correlating data mature, and as individuals in

Table 3. Host genes associated with variation in clinical presentation following chlamydial infection of humans

Gene	Correlation shown; system	Reference
Haptoglobin type E	active trachoma	[67]
Sickle cell trait HbAS	none	[67]
NLRP3	abdominal pain following *C. trachomatis* infection	[68]
miRNA-146A	none; genital tract	[68]
TLR-4 mutation	none; genital tract	[69]
MBL2	antibody response; *C. pneumoniae* infection	[70]
multiple SNPs in PRR's	trend toward relationship; tubal pathology	[71]
IL1-B, IL-1R	no association; tubal pathology	[72]
IL-8, CSF2, MMP9	association with trachomatous scarring	[73]
MMP9	scarring; ocular infection	[74]
TLR-4	pathogen accumulation; tubal factor infertility	[75]
MBL-low	susceptibility; tubal factor infertility	[75]
CCR5, TLR-2	none; tubal factor infertility	[75]
TLR-2 haplotype 1	reduced susceptibility; tubal pathology	[76]
MICA	host susceptibility; genital tract infection	[77]
IL-10, IFN-γ	immune response variation; tubal factor infertility	[78]
TNF-α, IL-10	severity of tubal damage; tubal factor infertility	[79]
HLA class I and II	chlamydial genital tract infection	[80]
HLA variants	recurrent infection	[81]

the field develop standardized metrics for integrating these data, increased clarity in these areas will emerge. It is anticipated that this field will move toward a clinically oriented integration of the host gene structure, chlamydial genes and genomes, the host microbiota and the health history of the patient, and that this integration will lead to more successful prediction of the patient prognosis following infection by *C. trachomatis* in the genital tract.

Acknowledgements

The Rockey Laboratory has been supported by PHS awards AI088540 and AI086469 and through internal funds at Oregon State University. We are grateful to the members of the Rockey laboratory for reading of the manuscript.

References

1 Ma B, Forney LJ, Ravel J: Vaginal Microbiome: Rethinking Health and Disease. Annu Rev Microbiol 2012;66:371–389.

2 Clarke IN: Evolution of *Chlamydia trachomatis*. Ann NY Acad Sci 2011;1230:E11–E18.

3 Stephens RS, Kalman S, Lammel C, Fan J, Marathe R, Aravind L, Mitchell W, Olinger L, Tatusov RL, Zhao Q, Koonin EV, Davis RW: Genome sequence of an obligate intracellular pathogen of humans: *Chlamydia trachomatis*. Science 1998;282:754–759.

4 Kalman S, Mitchell W, Marathe R, Lammel C, Fan J, Hyman RW, Olinger L, Grimwood J, Davis RW, Stephens RS: Comparative genomes of *Chlamydia pneumoniae* and *C. trachomatis*. Nat Genet 1999;21: 385–389.

5 Read TD, Brunham RC, Shen C, Gill SR, Heidelberg JF, White O, Hickey EK, Peterson J, Utterback T, Berry K, Bass S, Linher K, Weidman J, Khouri H, Craven B, Bowman C, Dodson R, Gwinn M, Nelson W, DeBoy R, Kolonay J, McClarty G, Salzberg SL, Eisen J, Fraser CM: Genome sequences of *Chlamydia trachomatis* MoPn and *Chlamydia pneumoniae* AR39. Nucleic Acids Res 2000;28:1397–1406.

6 Voigt A, Schofl G, Saluz HP: The *Chlamydia psittaci* genome: a comparative analysis of intracellular pathogens. PloS One 2012;7:e35097.

7 Read TD, Myers GS, Brunham RC, Nelson WC, Paulsen IT, Heidelberg J, Holtzapple E, Khouri H, Federova NB, Carty HA, Umayam LA, Haft DH, Peterson J, Beanan MJ, White O, Salzberg SL, Hsia RC, McClarty G, Rank RG, Bavoil PM, Fraser CM: Genome sequence of *Chlamydophila caviae* (*Chlamydia psittaci* GPIC): examining the role of niche-specific genes in the evolution of the Chlamydiaceae. Nucleic Acids Res 2003;31:2134–2147.

8 Azuma Y, Hirakawa H, Yamashita A, Cai Y, Rahman MA, Suzuki H, Mitaku S, Toh H, Goto S, Murakami T, Sugi K, Hayashi H, Fukushi H, Hattori M, Kuhara S, Shirai M: Genome sequence of the cat pathogen, *Chlamydophila felis*. DNA Res 2006;13:15–23.

9 Pannekoek Y, van der Ende A: Inclusion proteins of Chlamydiaceae. Drugs Today 2006;42(suppl A):65–73.

10 Byrne GI: *Chlamydia trachomatis* strains and virulence: rethinking links to infection prevalence and disease severity. J Infect Dis 2010;201(suppl 2):S126–S133.

11 Zhong G: *Chlamydia trachomatis* secretion of proteases for manipulating host signaling pathways. Front Microbiol 2011;2:14.

12 Clifton DR, Fields KA, Grieshaber SS, Dooley CA, Fischer ER, Mead DJ, Carabeo RA, Hackstadt T: A chlamydial type III translocated protein is tyrosine-phosphorylated at the site of entry and associated with recruitment of actin. Proc Natl Acad Sci USA 2004;101:10166–10171.

13 Jiwani S, Ohr RJ, Fischer ER, Hackstadt T, Alvarado S, Romero A, Jewett TJ: Chlamydia trachomatis Tarp cooperates with the Arp2/3 complex to increase the rate of actin polymerization. Biochem Biophys Res Commun 2012;420:816–821.

14 Schwarzenbacher R, Stenner-Liewen F, Liewen H, Robinson H, Yuan H, Bossy-Wetzel E, Reed JC, Liddington RC: Structure of the *Chlamydia* protein CADD reveals a redox enzyme that modulates host cell apoptosis. J Biol Chem 2004;279:29320–29324.

15 Fling SP, Sutherland RA, Steele LN, Hess B, D'Orazio SE, Maisonneuve J, Lampe MF, Probst P, Starnbach MN: CD8+ T cells recognize an inclusion membrane-associated protein from the vacuolar pathogen *Chlamydia trachomatis*. Proc Natl Acad Sci USA 2001;98:1160–1165.

16 Misaghi S, Balsara ZR, Catic A, Spooner E, Ploegh HL, Starnbach MN: *Chlamydia trachomatis*-derived deubiquitinating enzymes in mammalian cells during infection. Mol Microbiol 2006;61:142–150.

17 McLeod MP, Qin X, Karpathy SE, Gioia J, Highlander SK, Fox GE, McNeill TZ, Jiang H, Muzny D, Jacob LS, Hawes AC, Sodergren E, Gill R, Hume J, Morgan M, Fan G, Amin AG, Gibbs RA, Hong C, Yu XJ, Walker DH, Weinstock GM: Complete genome sequence of *Rickettsia typhi* and comparison with sequences of other rickettsiae. J Bacteriol 2004;186:5842–5855.

18 Andersson SG, Zomorodipour A, Andersson JO, Sicheritz-Ponten T, Alsmark UC, Podowski RM, Naslund AK, Eriksson AS, Winkler HH, Kurland CG: The genome sequence of *Rickettsia prowazekii* and the origin of mitochondria. Nature 1998;396: 133–140.

19 Fraser CM, Norris SJ, Weinstock GM, White O, Sutton GG, Dodson R, Gwinn M, Hickey EK, Clayton R, Ketchum KA, Sodergren E, Hardham JM, McLeod MP, Salzberg S, Peterson J, Khalak H, Richardson D, Howell JK, Chidambaram M, Utterback T, McDonald L, Artiach P, Bowman C, Cotton MD, Fujii C, Garland S, Hatch B, Horst K, Roberts K, Sandusky M, Weidman J, Smith HO, Venter JC: Complete genome sequence of *Treponema pallidum*, the syphilis spirochete. Science 1998;281:375–388.

20 Fadiel A, Eichenbaum KD, El Semary N, Epperson B: Mycoplasma genomics: tailoring the genome for minimal life requirements through reductive evolution. Front Biosci 2007;12:2020–2028.

21 Rockey DD: Unraveling the basic biology and clinical significance of the chlamydial plasmid. J Exp Med 2011;208:2159–2162.

22 Carlson JH, Whitmire WM, Crane DD, Wicke L, Virtaneva K, Sturdevant DE, Kupko JJ 3rd, Porcella SF, Martinez-Orengo N, Heinzen RA, Kari L, Caldwell HD: The *Chlamydia trachomatis* plasmid is a transcriptional regulator of chromosomal genes and a virulence factor. Infect Immun 2008;76:2273–2283.

23 Hacker J, Kaper JB: Pathogenicity islands and the evolution of microbes. Annu Rev Microbiol 2000;54: 641–679.

24 Song L, Carlson JH, Whitmire WM, Kari L, Virtaneva K, Sturdevant DE, Watkins H, Zhou B, Sturdevant GL, Porcella SF, McClarty G, Caldwell HD: Chlamydia trachomatis plasmid-encoded Pgp4 is a transcriptional regulator of virulence-associated genes. Infection and Immunity 2013;81:636–644.

25 Unemo M, Clarke IN: The Swedish new variant of *Chlamydia trachomatis*. Curr Opin Infect Dis 2011; 24:62–69.

26 Collingro A, Tischler P, Weinmaier T, Penz T, Heinz E, Brunham RC, Read TD, Bavoil PM, Sachse K, Kahane S, Friedman MG, Rattei T, Myers GS, Horn M: Unity in variety – the pan-genome of the Chlamydiae. Mol Biol Evol 2011;28:3253–3270.

27 Dobrindt U, Chowdary MG, Krumbholz G, Hacker J: Genome dynamics and its impact on evolution of *Escherichia coli*. Med Microbiol Immunol 2010;199: 145–154.

28 Dugan J, Rockey DD, Jones L, Andersen AA: Tetracycline resistance in *Chlamydia suis* mediated by genomic islands inserted into the chlamydial inv-like gene. Antimicrob Agents Chemother 2004;48:3989–3995.

29 Dugan J, Andersen AA, Rockey DD: Functional characterization of IScs605, an insertion element carried by tetracycline-resistant *Chlamydia suis*. Microbiology 2007;153:71–79.

30 Di Francesco A, Donati M, Rossi M, Pignanelli S, Shurdhi A, Baldelli R, Cevenini R: Tetracycline-resistant *Chlamydia suis* isolates in Italy. Vet Rec 2008; 163:251–252.

31 Suchland RJ, Sandoz KM, Jeffrey BM, Stamm WE, Rockey DD: Horizontal transfer of tetracycline resistance among *Chlamydia* spp. in vitro. Antimicrob Agents Chemother 2009;53:4604–4611.

32 Yuan Y, Zhang YX, Watkins NG, Caldwell HD: Nucleotide and deduced amino acid sequences for the four variable domains of the major outer membrane proteins of the 15 *Chlamydia trachomatis* serovars. Infect Immun 1989;57:1040–1049.

33 Lampe MF, Suchland RJ, Stamm WE: Nucleotide sequence of the variable domains within the major outer membrane protein gene from serovariants of *Chlamydia trachomatis*. Infect Immun 1993;61:213–219.

34 Beatty WL, Belanger TA, Desai AA, Morrison RP, Byrne GI: Tryptophan depletion as a mechanism of gamma interferon-mediated chlamydial persistence. Infect Immun 1994;62:3705–3711.

35 Roshick C, Wood H, Caldwell HD, McClarty G: Comparison of gamma interferon-mediated antichlamydial defense mechanisms in human and mouse cells. Infect Immun 2006;74:225–238.

36 Caldwell HD, Wood H, Crane D, Bailey R, Jones RB, Mabey D, Maclean I, Mohammed Z, Peeling R, Roshick C, Schachter J, Solomon AW, Stamm WE, Suchland RJ, Taylor L, West SK, Quinn TC, Belland RJ, McClarty G: Polymorphisms in *Chlamydia trachomatis* tryptophan synthase genes differentiate between genital and ocular isolates. J Clin Invest 2003; 111:1757–1769.

37 Belland RJ, Scidmore MA, Crane DD, Hogan DM, Whitmire W, McClarty G, Caldwell HD: *Chlamydia trachomatis* cytotoxicity associated with complete and partial cytotoxin genes. Proc Natl Acad Sci USA 2001;98:13984–13989.

38 Carlson JH, Hughes S, Hogan D, Cieplak G, Sturdevant DE, McClarty G, Caldwell HD, Belland RJ: Polymorphisms in the *Chlamydia trachomatis* cytotoxin locus associated with ocular and genital isolates. Infect Immun 2004;72:7063–7072.

39 Nelson DE, Crane DD, Taylor LD, Dorward DW, Goheen MM, Caldwell HD: Inhibition of chlamydiae by primary alcohols correlates with the strain-specific complement of plasticity zone phospholipase D genes. Infect Immun 2006;74:73–80.

40 Clifton DR, Dooley CA, Grieshaber SS, Carabeo RA, Fields KA, Hackstadt T: Tyrosine phosphorylation of the chlamydial effector protein Tarp is species specific and not required for recruitment of actin. Infect Immun 2005;73:3860–3868.

41 Carlson JH, Porcella SF, McClarty G, Caldwell HD: Comparative genomic analysis of *Chlamydia trachomatis* oculotropic and genitotropic strains. Infect Immun 2005;73:6407–6418.

42 Dean D, Suchland RJ, Stamm WE: Evidence for long-term cervical persistence of *Chlamydia trachomatis* by omp1 genotyping. J Infect Dis 2000;182: 909–916.

43 Rockey DD, Viratyosin W, Bannantine JP, Suchland RJ, Stamm WE: Diversity within inc genes of clinical *Chlamydia trachomatis* variant isolates that occupy non-fusogenic inclusions. Microbiology 2002;148: 2497–2505.

44 Suchland RJ, Jeffrey BM, Xia M, Bhatia A, Chu HG, Rockey DD, Stamm WE: Identification of concomitant infection with *Chlamydia trachomatis* IncA-negative mutant and wild-type strains by genomic, transcriptional, and biological characterizations. Infect Immun 2008;76:5438–5446.

45 Geisler WM, Suchland RJ, Rockey DD, Stamm WE: Epidemiology and clinical manifestations of unique *Chlamydia trachomatis* isolates that occupy nonfusogenic inclusions. J Infect Dis 2001;184:879–884.

46 Sturdevant GL, Kari L, Gardner DJ, Olivares-Zavaleta N, Randall LB, Whitmire WM, Carlson JH, Goheen MM, Selleck EM, Martens C, Caldwell HD: Frameshift mutations in a single novel virulence factor alter the in vivo pathogenicity of *Chlamydia trachomatis* for the female murine genital tract. Infect Immun 2010;78:3660–3668.

47 Tan C, Hsia RC, Shou H, Carrasco JA, Rank RG, Bavoil PM: Variable expression of surface-exposed polymorphic membrane proteins in in vitro-grown *Chlamydia trachomatis*. Cell Microbiol 2010;12: 174–187.

48 Kari L, Whitmire WM, Carlson JH, Crane DD, Reveneau N, Nelson DE, Mabey DC, Bailey RL, Holland MJ, McClarty G, Caldwell HD: Pathogenic diversity among *Chlamydia trachomatis* ocular strains in non-human primates is affected by subtle genomic variations. J Infect Dis 2008;197:449–456.

49 Jeffrey BM, Suchland RJ, Quinn KL, Davidson JR, Stamm WE, Rockey DD: Genome sequencing of recent clinical *Chlamydia trachomatis* strains identifies loci associated with tissue tropism and regions of apparent recombination. Infect Immun 2010;78:2544–2553.

50 Klint M, Fuxelius HH, Goldkuhl RR, Skarin H, Rutemark C, Andersson SG, Persson K, Herrmann B: High-resolution genotyping of *Chlamydia trachomatis* strains by multilocus sequence analysis. J Clin Microbiol 2007;45:1410–1414.

51 Wang Y, Skilton RJ, Cutcliffe LT, Andrews E, Clarke IN, Marsh P: Evaluation of a high resolution genotyping method for *Chlamydia trachomatis* using routine clinical samples. PloS One 2011;6:e16971.

52 Dean D: *Chlamydia trachomatis* today: treatment, detection, immunogenetics and the need for a greater global understanding of chlamydial disease pathogenesis. Drugs Today 2009;45(suppl B):25–31.

53 Pannekoek Y, Morelli G, Kusecek B, Morre SA, Ossewaarde JM, Langerak AA, van der Ende A: Multi locus sequence typing of Chlamydiales: clonal groupings within the obligate intracellular bacteria *Chlamydia trachomatis*. BMC Microbiol 2008;8:42.

54 Pedersen LN, Podenphant L, Moller JK: Highly discriminative genotyping of *Chlamydia trachomatis* using *omp1* and a set of variable number tandem repeats. Clin Microbiol Infect 2008;14:644–652.

55 Peuchant O, Le Roy C, Herrmann B, Clerc M, Bebear C, de Barbeyrac B: MLVA subtyping of genovar E *Chlamydia trachomatis* individualizes the Swedish variant and anorectal isolates from men who have sex with men. PloS One 2012;7:e31538.

56 Somboonna N, Wan R, Ojcius DM, Pettengill MA, Joseph SJ, Chang A, Hsu R, Read TD, Dean D: Hypervirulent *Chlamydia trachomatis* clinical strain is a recombinant between lymphogranuloma venereum (L₂) and D lineages. mBio 2011;2:e00045–00011.

57 Harris SR, Clarke IN, Seth-Smith HM, Solomon AW, Cutcliffe LT, Marsh P, Skilton RJ, Holland MJ, Mabey D, Peeling RW, Lewis DA, Spratt BG, Unemo M, Persson K, Bjartling C, Brunham R, de Vries HJ, Morre SA, Speksnijder A, Bebear CM, Clerc M, de Barbeyrac B, Parkhill J, Thomson NR: Whole-genome analysis of diverse *Chlamydia trachomatis* strains identifies phylogenetic relationships masked by current clinical typing. Nat Genet 2012;44:413–419, S411.

58 Gomes JP, Bruno WJ, Nunes A, Santos N, Florindo C, Borrego MJ, Dean D: Evolution of *Chlamydia trachomatis* diversity occurs by widespread interstrain recombination involving hotspots. Genome Res 2007;17:50–60.

59 Spaargaren J, Schachter J, Moncada J, de Vries HJ, Fennema HS, Pena AS, Coutinho RA, Morre SA: Slow epidemic of lymphogranuloma venereum L2b strain. Emerg Infect Dis 2005;11:1787–1788.

60 Albrecht M, Sharma CM, Reinhardt R, Vogel J, Rudel T: Deep sequencing-based discovery of the *Chlamydia trachomatis* transcriptome. Nucleic Acids Res 2010;38:868–877.

61 Jorgensen I, Valdivia RH: Pmp-like proteins Pls1 and Pls2 are secreted into the lumen of the *Chlamydia trachomatis* inclusion. Infect Immun 2008;76:3940–3950.

62 Joseph SJ, Didelot X, Gandhi K, Dean D, Read TD: Interplay of recombination and selection in the genomes of *Chlamydia trachomatis*. Biol Direct 2011;6:28.

63 Thalmann J, Janik K, May M, Sommer K, Ebeling J, Hofmann F, Genth H, Klos A: Actin re-organization induced by *Chlamydia trachomatis* serovar D – evidence for a critical role of the effector protein CT166 targeting Rac. PloS One 2010;5:e9887.

64 Gomes JP, Nunes A, Bruno WJ, Borrego MJ, Florindo C, Dean D: Polymorphisms in the nine polymorphic membrane proteins of *Chlamydia trachomatis* across all serovars: evidence for serovar Da recombination and correlation with tissue tropism. J Bacteriol 2006;188:275–286.

65 Bannantine JP, Griffiths RS, Viratyosin W, Brown WJ, Rockey DD: A secondary structure motif predictive of protein localization to the chlamydial inclusion membrane. Cell Microbiol 2000;2:35–47.

66 Dean D, Bruno WJ, Wan R, Gomes JP, Devignot S, Mehari T, de Vries HJ, Morre SA, Myers G, Read TD, Spratt BG: Predicting phenotype and emerging strains among *Chlamydia trachomatis* infections. Emerg Infect Dis 2009;15:1385–1394.

67 Savy M, Hennig BJ, Doherty CP, Fulford AJ, Bailey R, Holland MJ, Sirugo G, Rockett KA, Kwiatkowski DP, Prentice AM, Cox SE: Haptoglobin and sickle cell polymorphisms and risk of active trachoma in Gambian children. PloS One 2010;5:e11075.

68 Wang W, Stassen FR, Surcel HM, Ohman H, Tiitinen A, Paavonen J, de Vries HJ, Heijmans R, Pleijster J, Morre SA, Ouburg S: Analyses of polymorphisms in the inflammasome-associated NLRP3 and miR-NA-146A genes in the susceptibility to and tubal pathology of *Chlamydia trachomatis* infection. Drugs Today 2009;45(suppl B):95–103.

69 den Hartog JE, Lyons JM, Ouburg S, Fennema JS, de Vries HJ, Bruggeman CA, Ito JI, Pena AS, Land JA, Morre SA: TLR4 in *Chlamydia trachomatis* infections: knockout mice, STD patients and women with tubal factor subfertility. Drugs Today 2009;45(suppl B):75–82.

70 Rantala A, Lajunen T, Juvonen R, Bloigu A, Paldanius M, Silvennoinen-Kassinen S, Peitso A, Vainio
O, Leinonen M, Saikku P: Low mannose-binding
lectin levels and MBL2 gene polymorphisms associate with *Chlamydia pneumoniae* antibodies. Innate
Immunity 2011;17:35–40.

71 den Hartog JE, Ouburg S, Land JA, Lyons JM, Ito JI,
Pena AS, Morre SA: Do host genetic traits in the
bacterial sensing system play a role in the development of *Chlamydia trachomatis*-associated tubal pathology in subfertile women? BMC Infect Dis 2006;
6:122.

72 Murillo LS, Land JA, Pleijster J, Bruggeman CA,
Pena AS, Morre SA: Interleukin-1B (IL-1B) and
interleukin-1 receptor antagonist (IL-1RN) gene
polymorphisms are not associated with tubal pathology and *Chlamydia trachomatis*-related tubal factor
subfertility. Hum Reprod 2003;18:2309–2314.

73 Natividad A, Hull J, Luoni G, Holland M, Rockett K,
Joof H, Burton M, Mabey D, Kwiatkowski D, Bailey
R: Innate immunity in ocular *Chlamydia trachoma-
tis* infection: contribution of IL8 and CSF2 gene vari-
ants to risk of trachomatous scarring in Gambians.
BMC Med Genet 2009;10:138.

74 Natividad A, Cooke G, Holland MJ, Burton MJ, Joof
HM, Rockett K, Kwiatkowski DP, Mabey DC, Bailey
RL: A coding polymorphism in matrix metallo-
proteinase 9 reduces risk of scarring sequelae of ocu-
lar *Chlamydia trachomatis* infection. BMC Med
Genet 2006;7:40.

75 Laisk T, Peters M, Saare M, Haller-Kikkatalo K, Kar-
ro H, Salumets A: Association of CCR5, TLR2, TLR4
and MBL genetic variations with genital tract infections and tubal factor infertility. J Reprod Immunol
2010;87:74–81.

76 Karimi O, Ouburg S, de Vries HJ, Pena AS, Pleijster
J, Land JA, Morre SA: TLR2 haplotypes in the susceptibility to and severity of *Chlamydia trachomatis*
infections in Dutch women. Drugs Today 2009;
45(suppl B):67–74.

77 Mei B, Luo Q, Du K, Huo Z, Wang F, Yu P: Association of MICA gene polymorphisms with *Chlamydia
trachomatis* infection and related tubal pathology in
infertile women. Hum Reprod 2009;24:3090–3095.

78 Ohman H, Tiitinen A, Halttunen M, Paavonen
J, Surcel HM: Cytokine gene polymorphism and
Chlamydia trachomatis-specific immune responses.
Hum Immunol 2011;72:278–282.

79 Ohman H, Tiitinen A, Halttunen M, Lehtinen M,
Paavonen J, Surcel HM: Cytokine polymorphisms
and severity of tubal damage in women with Chlamydia-associated infertility. J Infect Dis 2009;199:
1353–1359.

80 Geisler WM, Tang J, Wang C, Wilson CM, Kaslow
RA: Epidemiological and genetic correlates of incident *Chlamydia trachomatis* infection in North
American adolescents. J Infect Dis 2004;190:1723–
1729.

81 Wang C, Tang J, Geisler WM, Crowley-Nowick PA,
Wilson CM, Kaslow RA: Human leukocyte antigen
and cytokine gene variants as predictors of recurrent
Chlamydia trachomatis infection in high-risk adolescents. J Infect Dis 2005;191:1084–1092.

Daniel D. Rockey
Department of Biomedical Sciences, College of Veterinary Medicine
Oregon State University
Corvallis, OR 97331–4804 (USA)
E-Mail rockeyd@orst.edu

Chapter 4

Black CM (ed): Chlamydial Infection: A Clinical and Public Health Perspective.
Issues Infect Dis. Basel, Karger, 2013, vol 7, pp 78–88 (DOI: 10.1159/000348753)

Chlamydia trachomatis: Molecular Testing Methods

Charlotte A. Gaydos

Division of Infectious Diseases, Johns Hopkins University, Baltimore, Md., USA

Abstract

Screening tests to detect *Chlamydia trachomatis* infections have advanced to permit the detection of nucleic acids from organisms. The development of these molecular assays that can detect and amplify the specific nucleic acids from the genes of *C. trachomatis* are called nucleic acid amplification tests (NAATs) and they have expanded the range of available specimen types to include noninvasive samples, as well as the more traditional invasive sample types. These new molecular tests have thereby drastically extended the transit time and conditions from the sample collection to testing in the laboratory. These highly sensitive and specific NAATs are now the primary tests used to screen for *C. trachomatis* infections. For screening purposes, CDC recommends vaginal swabs from women and urine from men as the sample types. These noninvasive specimen types are most suitable for screening applications since the specimen can be collected in multiple venues, without the requirement of pelvic or urogenital examinations. Vaginal swab specimens are less invasive than endocervical swabs. When women are given the choice, they often prefer them above urine collection. These specimen types have been shown to be equal in sensitivity to endocervical swabs and slightly better than urine specimens for the detection of *C. trachomatis*. Thus, the use of NAAT assays has the potential to improve screening rates of both symptomatic and asymptomatic individuals for detection of chlamydia infections.

Chlamydia trachomatis is the most commonly reported communicable disease in the USA, which infects mostly among adolescent and young adult females. The Centers for Disease Control and Prevention (CDC) estimates there are 3 million new cases each year [1]. Acute chlamydia infections often have no symptoms, leaving many cases untreated. However, the infection may progress to serious health outcomes including pelvic inflammatory disease, infertility, ectopic pregnancy and chronic pelvic pain. Untreated chlamydia in a pregnant woman can also infect her newborn. These sequelae are preventable since chlamydia infections are easily treated with antibiotics.

The CDC and the US Preventive Services Task Force and major medical professional organizations recommend an annual screening test for chlamydia for all sexually active adolescents and young women 25 years of age and under, for all pregnant women and for women at high risk of infection because of sexual risk behavior [2, 3]. CDC also recommends that previously infected women be rescreened 3 months after being treated for a chlamydia infection [2]. However, chlamydia screening remains an underutilized clinical preventive service with less that 50% of eligible women being screened every year [4].

Improvements in the molecular technology of screening tests holds promise for increasing screening rates and preventing consequences of untreated infections. The use of new molecular tests such as nucleic acid amplification tests (NAATs) allows chlamydia testing on vaginal and urine specimens, as well as more traditional samples, such as endocervical swabs for women, thereby avoiding invasive specimen collection procedures which require a speculum examination. Also, urine samples from men can now be tested rather than more invasive urethral swabs. CDC now recommends use of vaginal swabs for women and urine from men as the preferred sample for chlamydia screening [5, 6]. Use of such noninvasive sample types have expanded the types of venues in which screening can be conducted.

Another potential advance likely to increase screening rates in women is the use of self-collected vaginal specimens obtained by the patient [7]. Shown to be both effective and accurate in detecting chlamydia, research has indicated that self-collected vaginal swabs are well accepted by women and are highly sensitive and specific for chlamydia [8, 9]. In one study women reported they would be more likely to be screened for STDs if they could collect their own samples [7]. This chapter reviews the different types of tests, specimen types and venues for the detection of and screening for chlamydia.

Tests for *C. trachomatis* Screening

Diagnostic Methods – Chlamydia

Chlamydiae were originally detected following cultivation in cell culture but this has largely been replaced by nonculture assays. Culture for detection of chlamydiae in clinical specimens is now usually only performed by large laboratories. Historically, culture for chlamydia was the first relatively sensitive method for detecting the presence of organisms in cervical samples. Although originally chlamydia was grown in embryonated chicken eggs, growth and detection of chlamydia is now accomplished by staining of chlamydial inclusions grown in tissue culture cells [10]. *C. trachomatis* is a biosafety level 2 agent and should be handled appropriately, although it is not considered a particularly dangerous pathogen. The cell line most commonly used is McCoy cells, but other cell lines have been used (monkey kidney, HeLa and HEp-2). As culture is technically difficult and has been shown to be not as sensitive as

Table 1. Estimates of sensitivity and specificity for diagnostic tests for *C. trachomatis* in urogenital specimens

Diagnostic method	Sensitivity, %	Specificity, %
Tissue culture	70–85	100
Direct fluorescent antibody	80–85	>99
Enzyme immunoassay	53–76	95
Direct hybridization	65–83	99
Polymerase chain reaction		
Cervical swabs	89.7	99.4
Female urine	89.2	99.0
Male urine	90.3	98.4
Strand displacement amplification		
Cervical swabs	92.8	98.1
Female urine	80.5	98.4
Male urine	94.5	91.4
Male urethral swabs	94.6	94.2
Transcriptional mediated amplification		
Cervical swabs	94.2	97.6
Vaginal swabs	96.6–96.7	97.6–97.1
Female urine	94.7	98.9
Male urine	97.0	99.1
Male urethral	95.2	98.2
Real-time PCR		
Cervical swabs	80.9–87.7	99.4–99.7
Vaginal swabs	84.8–94.7	98.8–99.1
Female urine	92.6–95.7	99.2–99.5
Male urine	97.3–97.8	99.6–99.7
Male urethral	88.6–93.3	98.3–99.1

Sensitivities and specificities adapted from clinical trial data, package inserts and selected published papers.

previously thought, it is rarely used, except for sexual abuse cases and medicolegal matters [11]. Previous studies have indicated that culture sensitivity compared to molecular techniques can range from 50 to 100%, and is usually considered to average 85%, while specificity is considered to be 100% (table 1) [10]. Culture is only performed today by highly specialized research laboratories and some state public health laboratories, as well as by the CDC. If a local state laboratory does not offer chlamydia culture when it is desired, the local laboratory should seek the assistance of the CDC in locating the appropriate site.

Early nonculture assays, such as direct fluorescent antibody staining of direct patient material and enzyme immunoassays, have been replaced by molecular tests called NAATs [12], which are currently the tests of choice [6]. Infections detected by NAATs may be up to 80% higher than those found with the use of older technology. Enzyme immunoassays and direct probe hybridization assays are no longer recommended because of their inferior sensitivity (table 1) [6].

Several NAATs are available commercially. These include: polymerase chain reaction (PCR; Amplicor, Roche Molecular Diagnostics, Indianapolis, Ind., USA); strand displacement amplification (SDA; ProbeTec, Becton-Dickson Inc., Sparks, Md., USA); transcription-mediated amplification (TMA; Aptima Combo 2, GenProbe Inc., San Diego, Calif., USA), and real-time m2000 PCR (Abbott Molecular Diagnostics, Des Plains, Ill., USA; table 1) [10, 13–15].

These methods have been found to have excellent sensitivity for detection of *C. trachomatis*, usually well above 90%, in genital specimens and urine from adult men and women, while maintaining high specificity [12]. A new genetic variant of *C. trachomatis* was discovered in Sweden in 2006, which was found to have a mutation in the sequence of the cryptic plasmid, at the target site for Roche PCR, rendering the organism undetectable by this assay [16]. Recent data from Sweden reports that this variant is now responsible for 20–65% of all detected chlamydial infection in counties where PCR was used. So far, this variant appears to be limited primarily to Sweden with a few isolates being identified in Norway and Denmark. Spread of the variant in Sweden was associated with use of PCR as the NAAT for diagnosis of *C. trachomatis* infection. It has not yet been detected in the USA [17].

NAATs are currently recommended by CDC as the diagnostic assays of choice [6]. Point-of-care tests, which can be used in doctors' offices and potentially by trained healthcare workers, are not yet of sufficient sensitivity to be recommended, but new assays are under development. Such tests could eliminate the need for laboratory facilities and could be used in community settings [18].

Choice of Specimen Type for Screening
The specimens traditionally used have been cervical swabs for females and urethral swabs for males. However, due to the great increase in sensitivity and specificity of NAAT assays, less invasive samples such as urines for both females and males, as well as vaginal swabs for females, can be also used. CDC now recommends that for screening of asymptomatic women that vaginal swabs should be used, since they are slightly more sensitive than urine [6]. Three commercially available NAATs are FDA cleared for use with vaginal swabs collected either by clinicians or patients during a healthcare visit.

Vaginal swab specimens are less invasive than endocervical swabs and, when patients are given the choice, are often preferred over urine collection [9, 19–21]. Vaginal swabs have been successfully used previously for chlamydia screening in many research studies [8, 22–25]. Such samples can eliminate the necessity for a clinician-performed pelvic examination for asymptomatic women and may be cost saving, when a Pap test is not required [26]. These specimen types have been shown to be equal to endocervical swabs and slightly better than urine specimens for the detection of *C. trachomatis*. Furthermore, patients can perform self-collection without a loss in sensitivity as measured against clinician-collected vaginal swabs.

However, urine screening tests are often used in outreach screening programs. Testing urine for the presence of *C. trachomatis* has greatly enhanced expansion of screening programs and has shown to be widely acceptable to patients, providers and laboratory staff. However, collection, transport and processing of urine may sometimes result in leakage and spillage. Patients may also be reluctant to provide a urine specimen, as it is often associated with drug testing.

When pelvic examinations are being performed for symptoms or because a Pap test is required, the cervical swab is usually preferred as the sample type has been shown to have a slightly higher organism load for chlamydia [27]. Cervical specimens are also acceptable for NAAT testing in those settings that combine Pap and chlamydia testing from the same swab sample, such as with the use of liquid cytology media. Liquid cytology transport media are cleared by the FDA for several commercial assays. However, using liquid cytology samples may lead to testing of older women at low risk for infection. However, if an individual recommended for screening is not receiving a pelvic examination, clinicians should take advantage of the ease of obtaining a urine sample or a self-collected vaginal swab for amplification testing for chlamydia.

For males, the urine specimen is the sample of choice for the detection of chlamydia by NAAT assays rather than the more invasive urethral swab [5, 6]. Studies demonstrate that urine samples perform with higher sensitivity than urethral swabs. Culture of urethral swabs is no longer recommended.

Alternative Specimen Types
Rectal and pharyngeal specimens are important sample types for detection of chlamydia in men who have sex with men. These sample types have been demonstrated to perform well with NAAT assays and yield better results than culture, but are not cleared by the FDA [28, 29]. Thus, verification of test performance by individual laboratories before use is required. Eye specimens from infants or ocular samples from adults can be tested by NAATs; again, laboratories must perform their own verification studies. Although the commercially available NAATs have FDA clearance for use in genital sites (cervix, vagina, self-collected vaginal swabs and male urethra) and urine from adolescents and adults, none are currently approved for any site in children. Since no company has sought FDA clearance for such nongenital sites or for children, individual laboratories must perform independent verification for using amplification assays for testing such specimens for diagnostic purposes in order to remain Clinical Laboratories Improvement Amendments (CLIA) compliant [30]. NAATs are also becoming increasingly used for diagnostic assays for cases of sexual abuse [31].

Diagnostic Limitations
Because NAATS measure nucleic acids instead of live organisms, care should be taken in using NAATS for test-of-cure assays. Residual nucleic acid from cells rendered noninfective by antibiotics may still give a positive amplified test up to 3 weeks after

treatment, when the patient is actually cured of viable organisms due to residual DNA in cells [32]. Thus, clinicians should not use NAATS for test-of-cure until after at least 3 weeks. The CDC does not recommend a test-of-cure after treatment for chlamydia, however, some clinicians still prefer to retest after therapy. Because incidence studies have demonstrated that previous chlamydia infection increases one's probability of becoming reinfected [33], the CDC recommends that previously infected women be rescreened at 3 months after treatment for chlamydia [2].

Populations to Screen
The steadily increasing cases being reported to the CDC every year and expansion of funds for screening programs for chlamydia has resulted in recommendations by professional organizations and public health officials to screen all sexually active women <26 years of age yearly, or those ≥26 years with sexual risk factors [2]. The CDC and professional organizations also recommend screening pregnant women because of the possibility of the infant becoming infected during birth. Such infections are usually seen in the eyes of babies, but there are cases where the infant may also develop pneumonia caused by chlamydia several months later. Babies with suspected ocular infections may be screened by obtaining swabs of the conjunctiva and sending them to the laboratory for either culture, which is FDA cleared, or for molecular NAAT assays. NAATs are not cleared by the FDA for use in testing conjunctival swabs, but in practice the assays work well and have been reported to be used by research studies. Theoretically, the individual laboratory would have to perform a verification study to ascertain adequate performance for the particular laboratory [30].

No official recommendations exist for screening asymptomatic or symptomatic men but CDC guidance has been published [34]. Some public health officials believe that screening men should be recommended, but others believe more women should be screened first based on the availability of funds. Some cost-effectiveness modeling studies have reported that screening men may be an effective way to prevent chlamydia sequelae in women [35–37].

Use of Nucleic Acid Amplification Tests in Cases of Suspected Sexual Abuse
A recent multicenter study by Black et al. [31] evaluated the use of SDA and TMA using urine and genital swabs (vagina and urethra) compared to culture for diagnosis of *C. trachomatis* in children, 0–13 years of age. Cultures for chlamydia were performed at the laboratories of each center, according to their own standard protocols. The commercial NAAT tests were performed at the CDC (SDA and TMA). When NAAT results were compared by the specimen type, only one girl had a discrepant result for chlamydia (vaginal swab negative, urine positive). The sensitivity of vaginal culture for chlamydia was 39% in all 485 girls studied. However, the sensitivities of urine and vaginal swab NAATs were 100 and 85% in all female children, respectively, for detection of *C. trachomatis* [31].

These results of Black et al. [31] suggest that NAATs, specifically SDA and TMA, can be used for detection of *C. trachomatis* in girls being evaluated for suspected sexual abuse. Limitations apply for use of these assays because the prevalence of *C. trachomatis* in this population is low, and thus confirmatory testing with a different NAAT is necessary. One cannot extrapolate from these results to other NAATs, specifically PCR, or use in specimens other than vagina and urine in girls. No recommendations can be made for the use of these assays in prepubertal boys.

For routine genital samples from adults and sexually active adolescents being tested, confirmatory testing originally recommended by CDC is no longer recommended by CDC [38]. However, for cases of suspected sexual abuse, confirmatory testing by a second NAAT should be performed and the laboratory should use a newer 'second generation' NAAT with the highest possible sensitivity [39]. Although confirmatory testing with a different NAAT target may be problematic, as most laboratories only use one type of assay, one commercial NAAT (TMA) offers an alternate target confirmation assay that can be used on the same testing platform. Additional options include sending specimens to a reference laboratory for confirmation testing. The 2010 CDC STD Treatment Guidelines recommended that NAATs can be used to detect *C. trachomatis* in vaginal swabs and urine from girls being evaluated for suspected sexual abuse [2]. However, NAATs were not recommended for use in boys or extragenital specimens, since there are no data. Specimens collected from children for forensic applications should always be retained in the laboratory for purposes of additional testing.

Serology

The microimmunofluorescence serological test has been the gold standard test for the detection of antibody for chlamydia [40]. The assay is useful for population studies but is not used for the diagnosis of *C. trachomatis* in ocular or urogenital disease. It has, however, been widely used for the diagnosis of *C. pneumoniae*, a respiratory chlamydial pathogen. The older complementation fixation serological test has historically been used for the diagnosis of infections caused by the LGV serovars of chlamydia, as well as for the confirmation of *C. psittaci* infections. LGV is the etiologic agent of lymphogranuloma venereum and some public health officials favor using serological assays for confirming the classical form of LGV. It is not recommended for diagnosing LGV from rectal specimens. The complementation fixation test and most other commercially available serological assays measure antibody to lipopolysaccharide, which is an antigen common to all chlamydia and thus these serological assays cannot distinguish between antibodies from different species of chlamydia. The microimmunofluorescence assay can be used to distinguish antibody from different species.

Barriers to Chlamydia Screening
There are barriers to chlamydia urogenital infection screening for both clinicians and patients. For providers, there is lack of reimbursement for time required, lack of awareness that patients are sexually active and lack of knowledge that screening can be performed without a pelvic examination. For patients, there are issues with inability to pay copayment of the test, lack of knowledge of the asymptomatic nature, high prevalence and lack of knowledge about the possible adverse long-term reproductive effects of chlamydia infection.

Providers, who are reluctant or too busy to perform pelvic examinations to collect cervical swabs, now have the opportunity to screen women with either urine or vaginal swabs. Patients who fear pelvic examinations can now submit urine or a self-collected vaginal swab for screening and no longer have to submit to a pelvic examination. Use of self-collected samples for chlamydia testing may eliminate some of these barriers for screening. Education of clinicians and patients alike will assist in overcoming these barriers. Making testing available free of charge from novel internet or similar school health-based clinic programs may also remove financial barriers [41–43].

Implications for Public Health Policy and Screening Programs
Continued expansion of chlamydia screening may likely require a systematic outreach approach to specimen collection in multiple venues, such as schools, vans, health fairs and including the home for transport delivery to a testing laboratory by courier or standard mail services [21, 42, 43]. Self-obtained vaginal swabs appear to be the most appropriate specimen type for outreach screening or home collection based on discreet packaging, less restrictive postal requirements and the lack of association with drug testing. However, until FDA clearance has been granted to home collection of specimens for *C. trachomatis* testing, program and medical directors must consult with their local laboratory directors on such use to satisfy CLIA regulations for off-label procedures [30].

In conclusion, screening tests to detect *C. trachomatis* infections have advanced to permit the detection of DNA or RNA from nonliving bacteria, thus extending transit time and conditions from the moment of collection to testing in the laboratory. Development of tests that can detect and amplify the specific nucleic acids from the genes of *C. trachomatis* have expanded the range of specimen types to include noninvasive samples, as well as the more traditional invasive sample types. These highly sensitive and specific tests are collectively known as NAATs and are the primary tests used to screen for *C. trachomatis* infections. For screening purposes, CDC recommends vaginal swabs from women and urine from men as the sample types. These noninvasive specimen types are most suitable for screening applications since the specimen can be collected in multiple venues without the requirement of pelvic or urogenital examinations.

Vaginal swab specimens are less invasive than endocervical swabs and, when patients are given the choice, are often preferred over urine collection [9, 19, 20, 38].

These specimen types have been shown to be equal in sensitivity to endocervical swabs and slightly better than urine specimens for the detection of *C. trachomatis*. Until FDA clearance has been granted to home collection of specimens for *C. trachomatis* testing, program and medical directors must consult with their constituent laboratory directors on study design to satisfy CLIA regulations for off-label procedures.

References

1 Centers for Disease Control and Prevention: Sexually Transmitted Disease Surveillance, 2009. Atlanta, US Department of Health and Human Services, 2010.

2 Centers for Disease Control and Prevention: Sexually transmitted disease treatment guidelines 2010. www.cdc.gov/std/treatment/2010 (accessed December 2010).

3 US Preventive Services Task Force: Screening for chlamydial infection: U.S. Preventive Services Task Force recommendation statement. Ann Intern Med 2007;147:128–134.

4 National Committee for Quality Assurance. The State of Health Care Quality 2010: HEDIS Measures of Care, Washington, NCQA, 2010, pp 43–44.

5 Gaydos CA, Ferrero DV, Papp J: Laboratory aspects of screening men for *Chlamydia trachomatis* in the new millennium. Sex Tansmit Dis 2008;35(suppl): S45–S50.

6 APHL/CDC Panel Summary Reports: Laboratory Diagnostic Testing for *Chlamydia trachomatis* and *Neisseria gonorrhoeae*, Laboratory Diagnostic Testing for *Treponema pallidum*: Guidelines for the Laboratory Testing of STDs. http://www.aphl.org/aphl-programs/infectious/std/Pages/stdtestingguidelines.aspx/2009.

7 Wiesenfeld HC, Lowry DLB, Heine RP, Krohn MA, Bittner H, Kellinger K, Schultz M, Sweet RL: Self-collection of vaginal swabs for the detection of Chlamydia, gonorrhea, and trichomonas. Sex Transm Dis 2001;28:321–325.

8 Schachter J, Chernesky MA, Willis DE, Fine PM, Martin DH, Fuller D, Jordan JA, Janda WM, Hook EW III: Vaginal swabs are the specimens of choice when screening for *Chlamydia trachomatis* and *Neisseria gonorrhoeae*: results from a multicenter evaluation of the APTIMA assays for both infections. Sex Transmit Dis 2005;32:725–728.

9 Chernesky MA, Hook EW, Martin DH, Lane J, Johnson R, Jordan JA, Fuller D, Willis DE, Fine PM, Janda WM, Schachter J: Women find it easy and prefer to collect their own vaginal swabs to diagnose *Chlamydia trachomatis* or *Neisseria gonorrhoeae* infections. Sex Transmit Dis 2005;32:729–733.

10 Gaydos CA: Chlamydiae; in Spector S, Hodinka RL, Young SA, Wiedbrauk DL (eds): Clinical Virology Manual, ed 4. Washington, ASM Press, 2009, pp 630–640.

11 Hammerschlag MR, Guillen CD: Medical and legal implications of testing for sexually transmitted infections in children. Clin Microbiol Rev 2010;23:493–506.

12 Gaydos CA: Nucleic acid amplification tests for gonorrhea and chlamydia: practice and applications; in Zenilman JM, Moellering RC Jr (eds): Infectious Diseases Clinics of North America, ed 19. Philadelphia, Elsevier Saunders, 2005, pp 367–386.

13 Campbell LA, Kuo C-C, Gaydos CA: Chlamydial infections; in Detrick B, Hamilton RG, Folds JD (eds): Manual of Molecular and Clinical Laboratory Immunology, ed 7. Washington, ASM Press, 2006, pp 518–525.

14 Kuypers J, Gaydos CA, Peeling RW: Principles of laboratory diagnosis of STIs; in Holmes KK, Sparling PF, Stamm WE, Piot P, Wasserheit JN, Corey L, et al. (eds): Sexually Transmitted Diseases, ed 4. New York, MeGraw Hill, 2008, pp 937–957.

15 Gaydos CA, Cartwright CP, Colaninno P, Welsch J, Holden J, Ho SY, Webb EM, Anderson C, Bertuzis R, Zhang L, Miller T, Leckie G, Abravaya K, Robinson J: Performance of the Abbott RealTime CT/NG for the Detection of *Chlamydia trachomatis* and *Neisseria gonorrhoeae*. J Clin Microbiol 2010;48:3236–3243.

16 Ripa T, Nilsson PA: A *Chlamydia trachomatis* strain with a 377-bp deletion in the cryptic plasmid causing false-negative nucleic acid amplification tests. Sex Transmit Dis 2007;34:255–256.

17 Gaydos CA, Hardick A, Ramachandron P, Papp J, Steece R, Vanderpol B, Moncada J, Schachter J: Development of a specific PCR for detection of the new variant strain of *Chlamydia trachomatis* and surveillance in the United States. Sixth Meeting of the European Society for Chlamydia Research. Aarhus, 1–4 July, 2008, p 63.

18 Huppert JS, Hesse E, Gaydos CA: What's the point? How point-of-care sexually transmitted infection tests can impact infected patients. Point Care 2010;9: 36–46.

19 Hsieh Y-H, Howell MR, Gaydos JC, McKee JKT, Gaydos CA: Preference among female army recruits for use of self-administered vaginal swabs or urine to screen for *Chlamydia trachomatis* genital infections. Sex Trans Dis 2003;30:769–773.

20 Newman SB, Nelson MB, Gaydos CA, Friedman HB: Female prisoners' preference of collection methods for testing for *Chlamydia trachomatis* and *Neisseria gonorrhoeae* infection. Sex Trans Dis 2003;30:306–309.

21 Grasek AA, Secura GM, Allsworth JE, Madden T, Peipert JF: Home-screening compared with clinic-based screening for sexually transmitted infections. Obstet Gynecol 2010;115:745–752.

22 Schachter J, McCormick WM, Chernesky MA, Martin DH, Van Der Pol B, Rice P, Hook III EW, Stamm WE, Quinn TC, Chow JM: Vaginal swabs are appropriate specimens for diagnosis of genital tract infection with *Chalmydia trachomatis*. J Clin Microbiol 2003;41:3784–3789.

23 Hsieh Y-H, Howell MR, Gaydos JC, McKee JKT, Quinn TC, Gaydos CA: Preference among female army recruits for use of self-administered vaginal swabs or urine to screen for *Chlamydia trachomatis* genital infections. Sex Transmit Dis 2003;30:769–773.

24 Hoebe CJPA, Rademaker CW, Brouwers EEHG, Ter Waarbeek HLG, Van Bergan JEAM: Acceptibility of self-taken vaginal swabs and first-catch urine samples for the diagnosis of urogenital *Chlamydia trachomatis* and *Neisseria gonorrhoeae* with an amplified DNA assay in young women attending a public health sexually transmitted disease clinic. Sex Transmit Dis 2006;33:491–495.

25 Hobbs MM, Van Der Pol B, Totten P, Gaydos CA, Wald A, Warren T, Winer RL, Cook RL, Deal CD, Rogers E, Schachter J, Holmes KK, Martin DH: From the NIH: Proceedings of a workshop on the importance of self-obtained vaginal specimens for detection of sexually transmitted infections. Sex Tansmit Dis 2008;35:8–13.

26 Blake D, Maldeis N, Barnes MR, Hardick A, Quinn TC, Gaydos CA: Cost-effectiveness of screening strategies for *Chlamydia trachomatis* using cervical swabs, urine, and self-obtained vaginal swabs in a Sexually Transmitted Disease clinic setting. Sex Transm Dis 2008;35:649–655.

27 Michel CC, Sonnex C, Carne CA, White JA, Magbanua JPV, Nadala ECB, Lee HH: *Chlamydia trachomatis* load at matched anatomical sites: implications for screening strategies. J Clin Microbiol 2007;45:1395–1402.

28 Schachter J, Moncada J, Liska S, Shayevich C, Klausner JD: Nucleic acid amplification tests in the diagnosis of chlamydial and gonococcal infections of the oropharynx and rectum of men who have sex with men. Sex Tansmit Dis 2008;35:637–642.

29 Ota KV, Tamari IE, Smieja M, Jamieson F, Jones KE, Towns L, Juzkiw J, Richardson SE: Detection of *Neisseria gonorrhoeae* and *Chlamydia trachomatis* in pharyngeal and rectal specimens using the BD Probetec ET sustem, the Gen-Probe Aptima combo2 assay and culture. Sex Transm Infect 2009;85:182–186.

30 Clark RB, Lewinski MA, Leoffelholz MJ, Tibbetts RJ: Verification and validation of procedures in the clinical microbiology laboratory. Cumitech (ASM Press) 2009;31A:1–24.

31 Black CM, Driebe EM, Howard LA, Fajman NN, Sawyer MK, Girardet RG, Sautter RL, Greenwald E, Beck-Sague CM, Unger ER, Igietseme JU, Hammerschlag MR: Multicenter study of nucleic acid amplification tests for detection of *Chlamydia trachomatis* and *Neisseria gonorrhoeae* in children being evaluated for sexual abuse. Pediatr Infect Dis J 2009;28:1–6.

32 Gaydos CA, Crotchfelt KA, Howell MR, Kralian S, Hauptman P, Quinn TC: Molecular amplification assays to detect chlamydial infections in urine specimens from high school female students and to monitor the persistance of chlamydial DNA after therapy. J Infect Dis 1998;177:417–424.

33 Gaydos CA, Wright C, Wood BJ, Waterfield G, Hobson S, Quinn TC: *Chlamydia trachomatis* re-infection rates among female adolescents seeking rescreening in school-based health centers. Sex Tansmit Dis 2008;35:233–237.

34 US Centers for Disease Control and Prevention: Male chlamydia screening consultation, March 28–29, 2006, Meeting Report. http://www.cdc.gov/std/chlamydia/ChlamydiaScreening-males.pdf (accessed February 2011).

35 Blake DR, Quinn TC, Gaydos CA: Should asymptomatic men be included in chlamydia screening programs? Cost-effectiveness of chlamydia screening among male and female entrants to a national job training program. Sex Tansm Dis 2008;35:91–101.

36 Nevin RL, Shuping EE, Frick KD, Gaydos JC, Gaydos CA: Cost and effectiveness of chlamydia screening among male military recruits: Markov modeling of complications averted through notification of prior female partners. Sex Transm Dis 2008;35:705–713.

37 Gift TL, Gaydos CA, Kent CK, Marrazzo JM, Rietmeijer CA, Schillinger JA, Dunn EF: The program cost and cost-effectiveness of screening men for chlamydia to prevent pelvic inflammatory disease in women. Sex Tansm Dis 2008;35(suppl):S66–S75.

38 Schachter J, Chow JM, Howard H, Bolan G, Moncada J: Detection of *Chlamydia trachomatis* by nucleic acid amplification testing: our evaluation suggests that CDC-recommended approaches for confirmatory testing are ill-advised. J Clin Microbiol 2006;44:2512–2517.

39 Schachter J, Hook EW 3rd, Martin DH, Willis D, Fine P, Fuller D, Jordan J, Janda WM, Chernesky M: Confirming positive results of nucleic acid amplification tests (NAATs) for *Chlamydia trachomatis*: all NAATS are not created equal. J Clin Microbiol 2005; 43:1372–1373.

40 Wang SP, Kuo CC, Grayston JT: Formalinized *Chlamydia trachomatis* organisms as antigens in the micro-immunofluorescence test. J Clin Microbiol 1979; 10:259–261.

41 Gaydos CA, Wright C, Wood BJ, Waterfield G, Hobson S, Quinn TC: *Chlamydia trachomatis* reinfection rates among female adolescents seeking rescreening in school-based health centers. Sex Tansmit Dis 2008;35:233–237.

42 Gaydos CA, Barnes M, Aumakham B, Quinn N, Agreda P, Whittle P, Hogan T: Can E-technology through the Internet be used as a new tool to address the *Chlamydia trachomatis* epidemic by home samplng and vaginal swabs? Sex Tansmit Dis 2009;36: 577–580.

43 Joffe A, Reitmeijer CA, Chung S, Willard N, Chapin JB, Lloyd LV, Waterfield GA, Ellen JE, Gydos CA: Screening asymptomatic adolescent males for *Chlamydia trachomatis* in school-based health Centers using urine-based nucleic acid amplification tests. Sex Transm Dis 2008;35(suppl):S19–S23.

Charlotte A. Gaydos, MS, MPH, DrPH
Professor of Medicine, Division of Infectious Diseases, Johns Hopkins University
530 Rangos Building, 855 N. Wolfe Street
Baltimore, MD 21205 (USA)
E-Mail cgaydos@jhmi.edu

Black CM (ed): Chlamydial Infection: A Clinical and Public Health Perspective.
Issues Infect Dis. Basel, Karger, 2013, vol 7, pp 89–96 (DOI: 10.1159/000348757)

Treatment of *Chlamydia trachomatis* Infections

Margaret R. Hammerschlag

Division of Pediatric Infectious Diseases, Departments of Pediatrics and Medicine,
SUNY Downstate Medical Center, Brooklyn, N.Y., USA

Abstract

Treatment of patients with *Chlamydia trachomatis* infection prevents sexual transmission. Treatment of sexual partners of infected individuals will also prevent reinfection of the index case and subsequent transmission to other sexual partners. Prompt treatment of chlamydial infection, especially in women, also reduces complications including pelvic inflammatory disease. Treatment of pregnant women will prevent the transmission of infection to infants during delivery, which has resulted in a dramatic decrease of perinatally acquired chlamydial infection (conjunctivitis and pneumonia) in the USA. The introduction of highly specific nucleic acid amplification tests for detection of *C. trachomatis* coupled with the availability of effective single-dose antibiotic treatment has had a major impact on control of genital chlamydial infections. This chapter will review the current recommendations for the treatment of *C. trachomatis* infections.

Treatment of patients with *Chlamydia trachomatis* infection prevents sexual transmission. Treatment of sexual partners of infected individuals will also prevent reinfection of the index case and subsequent transmission to other sexual partners. Prompt treatment of chlamydial infection, especially in women, may reduce complications including pelvic inflammatory disease (PID), ectopic pregnancy and infertility, although the extent is still controversial [1–3]. Treatment of pregnant women prevents transmission of infection to infants during delivery, which has resulted in a dramatic decrease of perinatally acquired chlamydial infection (conjunctivitis and pneumonia) in the USA [1]. As the majority of individuals with genital chlamydial infection are asymptomatic, screening is the foundation of control in many populations.

Table 1. MIC of antimicrobial agents active against *C. trachomatis*

Antimicrobial agent	MIC, µg/ml
Tetracycline	0.25–0.5
Doxycycline	0.031–0.25
Azithromycin	0.06–2
Erythromycin	0.016–2
Clindamycin	2–16
Moxifloxacin	0.015–1
Ciprofloxacin	0.5–2
Ofloxacin	0.5–1
Levofloxacin	0.12–0.5
Sulfamethoxazole	0.5–4
Amoxicillin	0.5–10
Rifampin	0.005–0.25
Gentamicin	500
Vancomycin	1,000

From references 7–9.

Antimicrobial Susceptibility of *C. Trachomatis*

Although there are no standardized methods for in vitro susceptibility testing of *Chlamydia* spp., results have been largely consistent [4–8]. *C. trachomatis* is susceptible in vitro to a variety of antimicrobial agents, primarily those that act against protein and DNA synthesis including rifampin, tetracyclines, macrolides, quinolones, sulfonamides and clindamycin [4–9] (table 1). All Chlamydiae are constitutively resistant to aminoglycosides and glycopeptides (table 1). Chlamydiae have a Gram-negative envelope without detectable peptidoglycan; however, genomic analysis has revealed that *C. trachomatis* encodes for proteins forming a nearly complete pathway for the synthesis of peptidoglycan, including 3 penicillin-binding proteins, thus penicillin and amoxicillin have been found to have some activity in vitro [10, 11]. This has been called the chlamydial paradox or anomaly.

The intracellular location of *Chlamydia* spp. requires that antimicrobial agents need to achieve adequate intracellular penetration and concentration to be effective. Efficacy is generally defined by a minimal inhibitory concentration (MIC) of 1 µg/ml or less, but an antibiotic with an MIC of 0.1 µg/ml may not necessarily have greater microbiologic efficacy in vivo than one with an MIC of 1 µg/ml. Ciprofloxacin has MICs of 0.5–2 µg/ml [8]. Two treatment studies of *C. trachomatis* urethritis in men found that a 7-day course of ciprofloxacin at doses of 750 mg bid and 1,000 mg bid had microbiologic efficacies of only 55 and 72%, respectively [12]. In contrast, levofloxacin has reported MICs of 0.12–0.5 µg/ml; one study of 500 mg daily for 7 days for treatment of *C. trachomatis* urethritis had a microbiologic efficacy of 92% [12].

Although resistance to quinolones and rifamycins can be induced in vitro by serial passage in subinhibitory concentrations of antibiotics [13–15], antibiotic resistance to *C. trachomatis* appears to be very uncommon in vivo. The number of passages needed to select for resistant mutants varied by strain and antibiotic. Point mutations for quinolone resistance were detected in both DNA gyrase and topoisomerase IV genes [13, 14]. The role of antimicrobial resistance in treatment failures or persistent infection is not clear. The potential of the organism to develop antimicrobial resistance in vivo has not been well studied, mostly limited to a few case reports that suggested that resistance was a possible cause of clinical treatment failure; however, the possible mechanisms of resistance were not well defined [5, 16]. In 2000, Somani et al. [17] described multidrug resistance to doxycycline, azithromycin and ofloxacin in *C. trachomatis* isolates from 3 patients, 2 of which were clinical and microbiologic failures, the third patient's infection being resolved despite resistance in vitro. They did not look for possible resistance-associated mutations. Misyurina et al. [18], from St. Petersburg, Russia, reported high level macrolide resistance in 4 clinical isolates of *C. trachomatis* associated with mutations in the 23SrRNA and L22 genes. The relationship to treatment and outcome were not clear as no information were provided on the clinical courses of these patients. More recently, Bhengraj et al. [19] reported identifying isolates with decreased susceptibility to azithromycin and doxycycline from 9 of 21(43%) women with recurrent *C. trachomatis* infection in New Delhi, India. The women presented with cervicitis, PID and infertility. The MICs for azithromycin and doxycycline ranged from 0.12 to 8 µg/ml. There was no consistent association of high MIC with previous treatment with either drug. It is possible that this may represent the baseline susceptibilities of *C. trachomatis* isolates circulating in this community. Neither of these studies attempted to look for any specific mutations. *C. trachomatis* appears to display what is called heterotypic resistance in vitro, meaning that the population contains both sensitive and resistant organisms. Studies have suggested that approximately 1% of the population will demonstrate resistance [17].

Most recurrent *C. trachomatis* infections result from reinfection from an untreated partner or new infection from a new sexual partner [1]. Studies examining the in vitro susceptibilities of recent clinical isolates from patients with *C. trachomatis* infection seen in the USA and Israel did not reveal any resistant organisms [20, 21]. A large survey of *C. trachomatis* isolates from patients with trachoma did not detect development of macrolide or doxycycline resistance 18 months after 4 biannual community-wide distributions of azithromycin [22]. These treatment distributions for trachoma control involved hundreds of individuals ≥1 year of age receiving a single dose of azithromycin, 20mg/kg in children or 1 g in adults, twice a year, which could conceivably provide selective pressure which might enable expansion of resistant clones of *C. trachomatis*. The communitywide azithromycin exposure with treatment of chlamydial genital infections is significantly less than the mass treatments required for control of trachoma.

Table 2. Treatment of uncomplicated *C. trachomatis* infection in adult and adolescent men and women

Recommended regimens
Azithromycin 1 g orally in a single dose
or
Doxycycline 100 mg orally twice a day for 7 days
Alternative regimens
Erythromycin base 500 mg orally four times a day for 7 days
or
Erythromycin ethylsuccinate 800 mg orally four times a day for 7 days
or
Levofloxacin 500 mg orally once daily for 7 days
or
Ofloxacin 300 mg orally twice a day for 7 days

Adapted from Workowski et al. [1].

Determining antibiotic resistance in *C. trachomatis* is hampered by the lack of a standardized in vitro assay. Currently very few laboratories are performing chlamydia culture, nucleic acid amplification tests (NAATs) are now the standard for the diagnosis of *C. trachomatis* genital infections. Possible mutations associated with antibiotic resistance in *C. trachomatis* are not well characterized and there are no standardized molecular tests for these mutations.

Treatment of *C. trachomatis* Infections in Adults and Adolescents

Because of the long life cycle of *C. trachomatis*, 48–72 h depending on biovar and strain, treatment has in the past required multiple dose treatment regimens. For decades, 7-day courses of doxycycline and erythromycin were the standard treatment. The need for multiple dose regimens has raised concerns about the impact on compliance. The introduction of azithromycin with its long half-life in tissue has allowed for single-dose treatment of genital *C. trachomatis* infections [1]. A meta-analysis of 12 randomized clinical trials comparing single-dose azithromycin to a 7-day course of doxycycline found a rate of microbiologic eradication of 97% for azithromycin and 98% for doxycycline [23]. Both drugs also had similar tolerability. Currently, the Centers for Disease Control and Prevention (CDC) recommends either single-dose azithromycin or a 7-day course of doxycycline as the first-line regimens for the treatment of uncomplicated genital *C. trachomatis* infection in adolescent and adult men and women [1] (table 2). Alternative regimens include a 7-day course of erythromycin base or ethylsuccinate. Erythromycin has a higher rate of gastrointestinal side effects than either azithromycin or doxycycline, which may contribute to the lower efficacy seen in a number of studies. Levofloxacin and ofloxacin are also listed as alternative treatment regimens; however, they are more expensive and require multiple dosing which offers no advantages over the first-line recommendations. Data on other quinolones are very limited. In a recent study comparing oral moxifloxacin (400 mg orally daily for 14 days) to levofloxacin (500 mg daily for 14 days) plus metronidazole for the treatment of uncomplicated PID, moxifloxacin eradicated *C. trachomatis* from 8 of 8 (100%) women compared to 10 of 12 (83.3%) who were treated with levofloxacin [24]. Moxifloxacin does not have an indication for treatment of genital *C. trachomatis* infections.

Test-of-cure (repeat testing 3–4 weeks after completion of therapy) is not generally recommended for individuals treated with a recommended or alternative regimen. However, if there are concerns about compliance, persisting symptoms or reinfection, repeat testing is indicated. Repeat testing using NAATs after completion of treatment may not be accurate as chlamydial DNA can persist for 21 days or longer.

Treatment of Pregnant Women

Screening and treatment of pregnant women is the most effective way to prevent transmission to the infant and subsequent infection, including conjunctivitis and pneumonia [1]. The CDC recommends repeat testing of pregnant women, preferably by NAAT, to document eradication 3 weeks after treatment. Doxycycline and quinolones are contraindicated for use in pregnancy. Single-dose azithromycin has been found to be both safe and effective in pregnant women [25], although few studies have followed the infants after delivery. The CDC also recommends amoxicillin as a first-line treatment regimen [1] (table 3). Amoxicillin has been demonstrated to be more effective and better tolerated than erythromycin, which was the recommended regimen for use in pregnancy for many years [1, 25].

Pregnant women treated for chlamydial infection during the first trimester should have test-of-cure, and should also be retested 3 months later.

Treatment of Lymphogranuloma Venereum

Lymphogranuloma venereum (LGV) is a systemic, invasive chlamydia infection caused by the *C. trachomatis* serovars L1, L2 or L3. Most LGV infection seen in Europe and the USA has been due to L2 strains. If not treated early and appropriately, LGV can lead to serious sequelae in men and women, including colorectal fistulas, strictures and elephantiasis. Unlike uncomplicated genital infection due to trachoma biovar strains of *C. trachomatis*, treatment of LGV requires a prolonged course of therapy. Published studies have demonstrated persistent *C. trachomatis* RNA in rectal samples from patients with LGV proctocolitis after 2 weeks of doxycycline,

Table 3. Treatment of *C. trachomatis* infection in pregnant women

Recommended regimens
    Azithromycin 1 g orally in a single dose
    or
    Amoxicillin 500 mg orally three times a day for 7 days
Alternative regimens
    Erythromycin base 500 mg orally four times a day for 7 days
    or
    Erythromycin base 250 mg orally four times a day for 14 days
    or
    Erythromycin ethylsuccinate 800 mg orally four times a day for 7 days
    or
    Erythromycin ethylsuccinate 400 mg orally four times a day for 14 days

Adapted from Workowski et al. [1].

Table 4. Treatment of LGV

Recommended regimen
    Doxycycline 100 mg orally twice a day for 21 days
Alternative regimen
    Erythromycin base 500 mg orally four times a day for 21 days

Adapted from Workowski et al. [1].

whereas in comparison, *C. trachomatis* DNA was undetectable after 7 days of treatment in patients with proctitis due to trachoma biovar strains [26]. Although 21-day treatment with doxycycline appears to be very effective, there have been reports of failure, usually in men coinfected with HIV [27]. Data on the use of other antibiotics, including azithromycin and quinolones, are limited to anecdotal reports, although in vitro susceptibilities against *C. trachomatis* suggest that they would be effective (table 1). Regimens of azithromycin used have included a single 1-gram dose and 1 gram weekly for 3 weeks [1, 28]. The patient reported by Méchaï et al. [27], who failed 3 weeks of doxycycline, was successfully treated with 400 mg moxifloxacin for 10 days.

The CDC recommends doxycycline, 100 mg orally twice daily for 21 days as the first line treatment regimen. Erythromycin base, 500 mg orally 4 times daily for 21 days is the alternative regimen (table 4).

References

1 Workowski KA, Berman S, Centers for Disease Control and Prevention: 2010 Sexually transmitted diseases treatment guidelines, 2010. MMWR Recomm Rep 2010;59:1–110.

2 Oakshott P, Kerry S, Aghaizu A, Atherton H, Hay S, Taylor-Robinson, Simms I, Hay P: Randomised controlled trial of screening for *Chlamydia trachomatis* to prevent pelvic inflammatory disease: the POPI (prevention of pelvic infection) trial. BMJ 2010; 340:c1642.

3 Gottlieb SL, Berman SM, Low N: Screening and treatment to prevent sequelae in women with *Chlamydia trachomatis* genital infection: how much do we know? J Infect Dis 2010;201(S2):S156–S167.

4 Suchland RJ, Geisler WM, Stamm WE: Methodologies and cell lines used for antimicrobial susceptibility testing of *Chlamydia* spp. Antimicrob Agents Chemother 2002;47:636–642.

5 Sandoz KM, Rockey DD: Antibiotic resistance in Chlamydiae. Future Microbiol 2010;5:1427–1442.

6 Wang SA, Papp JR, Stamm WE, Peeling RW, Martin DH, Holmes KK: Evaluation of antimicrobial resistance and treatment failures for *Chlamydia trachomatis*: a meeting report. J Infect Dis 2005;191:917–923.

7 Senn L, Hammerschlag MR, Greub G: Therapeutic approaches to *Chlamydia* infections. Expert Opin Pharmacother 2005;6:1–10.

8 Schachter J, Stephens RS: Biology of *Chlamydia trachomatis;* in Holmes KK, Sparling PF, Stamm WE, Piot P, Wasserheit JN, Cory L, Cohen M, Watts H (eds): Sexually Transmitted Diseases, ed 4. New York, McGraw Hill, 2008, pp 555–574.

9 Bébéar CM, de Barbeyrac B, Pereyre S, Renaudin H, Clerc M, Bébéar C: Activity of moxifloxacin against urogenital mycoplasmas *Ureaplasma* spp., *Mycoplasma hominis,* and *Mycoplasma genitalium* and *Chlamydia trachomatis*. Clin Microbiol Infect 2008; 14:801–805.

10 Rockey DD, Lenart J, Stephens RS: Genome sequencing and our understanding of chlamydiae. Infect Immun 2000;68:5473–5479.

11 Ghuysen JM, Goffin C: Lack of cell wall peptidoglycan versus penicillin sensitivity: new insights into the chlamydial anomaly. Antimicrob Agents Chemother 1999;43:2339–2344.

12 Stamm WE: *Chlamydia trachomatis* infections in the adult; in Holmes KK, Sparling PF, Stamm WE, Piot P, Wasserheit JN, Cory L, Cohen M, Watts H (eds): Sexually Transmitted Diseases, ed 4. New York, McGraw Hill, 2008, pp 575–594.

13 Dessus-Babus S, Bébéar CM, Charron A, Bébéar C, de Barbeyrac B: Sequencing of gyrase and topoisomerase IV quinolones sequence-determining regions of *Chlamydia trachomatis* and characterization of quinolones resistant mutants obtained in vitro. Antimicrob Agents Chemother 1998;42:2474–2481.

14 Morrissey I, Salman H, Bakker S, Farrell D, Bébéar CM, Ridgway G: Serial passage of *Chlamydia* spp. in subinhibitory fluoroquinolone concentrations. J Antimicrob Chemother 2002;49:757–761.

15 Kutlin A, Kohlhoff S, Roblin P, Hammerschlag MR, Riska P: Emergence of resistance to rifampin and rifalazil in *Chlamydophila pneumoniae* and *Chlamydia trachomatis*. Antimicrob Agents Chemother 2005; 49:903–907.

16 Jones RB, Van Der Pol B, Martin DH, Shepard MK: Partial characterization of *Chlamydia trachomatis* isolates resistant to multiple antibiotics. J Infect Dis 1990;162:1309–1315.

17 Somani J, Bhullar VB, Workowski KA, Farshy CE, Black CM: Multiple drug- resistant *Chlamydia trachomatis* associated with clinical treatment failure. J Infect Dis 2000;181:1421–1427.

18 Misyurina OY, Chipitsyna EV, Finashutina YP, Lazarev VN, Akopian TA, Savicheva AM, Govorun VM: Mutations in a 23S rRNA gene of *Chlamydia trachomatis* associated with resistance to macrolides. Antimicrob Agents Chemother 2004;48:1347–1349.

19 Bhengraj AR, Vardhan H, Srivastava P, Salhan S, Mittal A: Decreased susceptibility to Azithromycin and Doxycycline in clinical isolates of *Chlamydia trachomatis* obtained from recurrently infected female patients in India. Chemotherapy 2010;56:371–377.

20 Rice RJ, Bhullar V, Mitchell SH, Bullard J, Knapp JS: Susceptibilities of *Chlamydia trachomatis* isolates causing uncomplicated female genital tract infections and pelvic inflammatory disease. Antimicrob Agents Chemother 1995;39:760–762.

21 Samra Z, Rosenberg S, Soffer Y, Dan M: In vitro susceptibility of recent clinical isolates of *Chlamydia trachomatis* to macrolides and tetracyclines. Diagn Microbiol Infect Dis 2001;39:177–179.

22 Hong KC, Schachter J, Moncada J, Zhou Z, House J, Lietman TM: Lack of macrolide resistance in *Chlamydia trachomatis* after mass azithromycin distributions for trachoma. Emerg Infect Dis 2009;15:1088–1090.

23 Lau C-Y, Qureshi AK: Azithromycin versus doxycycline for genital chlamydial infections: a meta-analysis of randomized clinical trials. Sex Transm Dis 2002;29:497–502.

24 Judlin P, Liao Q, Liu Z, Reimitz, Hample B, Arvis P: Efficacy and safety of moxifloxacin in uncomplicated pelvic inflammatory disease: the MONALISA study. BJOG 2010;117:1475–1484.

25 Pitsouni E, Iavazzo C, Athtanasiou S, Falagas M: Single-dose azithromycin versus erythromycin or amoxicillin for *Chlamydia trachomatis* infection during pregnancy: a meta-analysis of randomized controlled trials. Int J Antimicrob Agents 2007;30: 213–221.

26 de Vries HJC, Smelov V, Middleburg JG, Pleijster J, Speksnijder AG, Morré SA: Delayed microbial cure of lymphogranuloma venerum proctitis with doxycycline treatment. Clin Infect Dis 2009;48:e53–e56.

27 Méchaï F, de Barbaeyrac D, Aoun O, Mérens A, Imbert P, Rapp C: Doxycycline failure in lymphogranuloma venerum. Sex Transm Infect 2010;86:278–279.

28 Nieuwenhuis RF, Ossewaarde JM, van der Meijden WI, Neumann HAM: Unusual presentation of early lymphogranuloma venereum in an HIV-1 infected patient: effective treatment with 1 g azithromycin. Sex Transm Infect 2003;79:453–455.

Margaret R. Hammerschlag, MD
Division of Infectious Diseases, Department of Pediatrics
SUNY Downstate Medical Center
450 Clarkson Avenue, Brooklyn, NY 11203-2098 (USA)
E-Mail mhammerschlag@downstate.edu

Black CM (ed): Chlamydial Infection: A Clinical and Public Health Perspective.
Issues Infect Dis. Basel, Karger, 2013, vol 7, pp 97–114 (DOI: 10.1159/000348759)

The Immunologic Response to Urogenital Infection

Raymond M. Johnson[a] · William Geisler[b]

[a]Microbiology and Immunology, Division of Infectious Diseases, Indiana University School of Medicine, Indianapolis, Ind., and [b]Department of Medicine, Division of Infectious Diseases, The University of Alabama at Birmingham, Birmingham, Ala., USA

Abstract

At the level of the herd (nations), the epidemic of *Chlamydia trachomatis* genital tract infections has not been controlled despite medical interventions including screening, treatment and partner management programs. However, at the level of the individual it is clear that the host immune response of humans and animals is capable of clearing infection, or at least controlling it asymptomatically at a level below that detectable with current diagnostic assays. Aggressive chlamydia screening and treatment programs appear to be counterproductive for reducing the incidence of disease, likely due to a detrimental effect on herd immunity. The unintentional demonstration of herd immunity revealed by unsuccessful antibiotic-based public health strategies offers a hopeful glimpse into possibilities for future immunologic/vaccine-based interventions. A key to successful implementation of a vaccine-based strategy will be understanding the immunologic goal of vaccination, i.e. the parameters that define a protective host immune response. In this chapter, we will examine what is currently known about the immune response to genital chlamydial infections based on data from experimental animal models and limited human studies.

Human Immune Response to Genital *Chlamydia trachomatis* Infection

In contrast to extensive data on the host immune responses elicited in animals during chlamydial infections (including clearance mechanisms), knowledge of immune responses to *C. trachomatis* infection and immune mechanisms mediating protective immunity are rather limited in humans. Because of ethical considerations, most human studies have evaluated immune responses at the time a patient is diagnosed with chlamydia, but have not performed repeated immune measures in patients with untreated infection that would provide more insight into the natural history of chlamydia and immune mechanisms mediating clearance. Some studies have demonstrated immune responses in patients with current genital chlamydial infections that were not *C. trachomatis* specific (i.e. not measured in vitro in response to challenge with *C. trachomatis* antigens), such as changes in genital mucosal concentrations of select cytokines [1–3], as well as increases in urethral polymorphonuclear cell counts [4] and cervical T cell but not B cell phenotypes [5]. A major limitation of many of these studies is that other potential pathogens (e.g. *Herpes simplex* virus, *Mycoplasma*, *Ureaplasma*, etc.) could also induce nonspecific immune responses and may not have been tested for or controlled for in the studies. Other studies have demonstrated *C. trachomatis*-specific immune responses during genital chlamydial infections, such as detection of: (1) serum and/or genital mucosal antibodies (mainly IgA and IgG) to *C. trachomatis* elementary bodies (EBs) or specific proteins (e.g. MOMP, PGP-3 and heat shock proteins, HSPs) [1, 2, 6, 7] and (2) systemic and mucosal lymphoproliferative (LP) responses of peripheral blood mononuclear cells (PBMCs) to *C. trachomatis* EBs or specific proteins, e.g. MOMP and HSPs [1, 8, 9]. However, most studies of *C. trachomatis*-specific immune responses have not correlated these responses with a clinical correlate of protective immunity, e.g. decreased risk for incident or recurrent chlamydia, in part due to a lack of large well-characterized human cohorts with clinical correlates of protective immunity.

Do humans develop protective immunity to *C. trachomatis* and what are the immune mechanisms mediating protection? Chlamydial reinfection within several months after treatment is common (about 10–20%) [10, 11], suggesting that some humans do not develop complete protective immunity. Yet other at-risk individuals do not get reinfected, likely due to some degree of protective immunity, a notion supported by epidemiological and natural history studies. Studies of persons with prior chlamydia or a high likelihood (e.g. commercial sex workers) show reduced risk of reinfection [12, 13]. Limited studies of the natural history of untreated chlamydia in humans have demonstrated that up to 28% of chlamydia-infected persons have spontaneous clearance of infection within several weeks of an initial screening test (i.e. before they receive treatment), and approximately 50% have cleared infection by 1 year [14]. These studies support the notion that some humans develop protective immunity to *C. trachomatis*, yet studies on the underlying immune mechanisms are sparse.

Human data that are available, as in animal models, suggest that CD4 T cells and Th1 responses are important. In a longitudinal study of host immune responses in commercial sex workers in Nairobi who were at high risk for chlamydia, Cohen et al. [8] reported that select PBMC IFN-γ responses to *C. trachomatis* HSP60 measured in subjects at baseline correlated with protection against incident chlamydial infections. Debattista et al. [9] reported that women accessing an Australian sexual health clinic who had PID or a history of multiple chlamydial infections had a reduced PBMC IFN-γ response to *C. trachomatis* HSP60 compared with women with only a single chlamydial infection or those with infertility due to endometriosis. Agrawal et al. [1] evaluated differences in host immune responses in female subjects with assumed primary versus recurrent genital chlamydial infections (based on absence vs. presence of serum *C. trachomatis* IgG, respectively) and found cervical LP responses to *C. trachomatis* HSP10 were higher in recurrent infection while LP responses to MOMP were higher in primary infection; another key finding was that IFN-γ levels were higher in cervical washes of women with recurrent infection than primary infection. Finally, a study by Wang et al. [15] evaluated immunogenetic determinants predicting recurrent chlamydia in adolescents enrolled in the multicenter longitudinal study 'Reaching for Excellence in Adolescent Care and Health' and found that females without an IL-10 gene promoter variant (promoter positions –1082, –819 and –592) had more recurrent chlamydial infections, and that this variant correlated with lower endocervical IL-10 levels (not *C. trachomatis* specific). Other studies have also linked select genetic variants to chlamydia complications (e.g. pelvic inflammatory disease and infertility) [16–19].

Data on the contribution of the humoral arm of the adaptive immune response towards protective immunity to *C. trachomatis* infection in humans are also sparse but suggest that the humoral response may contribute. Brunham et al. [20] reported chlamydia-infected women with anti-*C. trachomatis* IgA in endocervical secretions shed fewer infectious *Chlamydiae* than women without anti-chlamydial IgA, but the correlation was not observed with serum antibodies. Similarly, Cunningham et al. [21] reported that the presence of genital anti-*C. trachomatis* IgA appeared to expedite chlamydia clearance in women following treatment, but serum IgG did not appear to influence clearance. However, the Cohen et al. [8] study discussed above found that neither cervical nor serum antibodies against *C. trachomatis* EBs and HSP60 were associated with a decrease in incident chlamydial infections.

A major limitation of many studies of immune responses predicting protective immunity to *C. trachomatis* infection was generalizability of the patient population studied. Some studies included HIV-infected persons or those with multiple prior sexually transmitted infections, which could have confounded immune responses. Also, differences in the race/ethnicity of the patient populations could influence the generalizability of the observations beyond the patient populations studied. In summary, there are a limited number of studies of host immune responses in genital *C. trachomatis* infections in humans, and studies on *C. trachomatis*-specific immune responses that influence protective immunity are sparse but suggest some humans do develop protective cellular and/or humoral immune responses.

Immunological Data from Animal Models of Genital *Chlamydia* Infection

The Animal Models
Animal models are essential for understanding host defense mechanisms because they allow experimental host manipulation to definitively test protective immunity

hypotheses. The major animal models for *C. trachomatis* urogenital infections are the *C. muridarum* mouse model, infection of mice with human *C. trachomatis* strains, and the *C. caviae* guinea pig model. The mouse models bring with them affordability, a reasonable reproduction of the natural human genital tract infection, including development of hydrosalpinx and infertility, and a wealth of reagents including knockout mice. The guinea pig model, while somewhat limited in reagents and genetic tools, is a reasonable reproduction of the human infection including development of hydrosalpinx with the additional advantage of sexual transmission of infection between male and female guinea pigs [22, 23].

Information gleaned from animal models is predisposed to misgivings about extrapolation to humans. This is a valid scientific concern, and a careful assessment of the animal model versus the human host is appropriate when interpreting animal model data. Use of human *C. trachomatis* strains rather than *C. muridarum* in the mouse model avoids issues related to the genetic drift that occurred in the million years since they diverged from a common ancestor, but brings with it liabilities related to species-specific adaptations that occurred in the same timeframe. Additionally, animal homologs for the human HLA-A/B/C/D antigen presentation molecules are also evolutionarily divergent, making it highly unlikely that 8–14 amino acid T cell epitopes identified in an animal model would have any relevance for human immunity. However, because many or possibly most potential *Chlamydia* T cell epitopes are sequestered in the inclusion body, identification of *Chlamydia* proteins whose roles in pathogen-host interactions make them accessible to host cell antigen processing pathways is species-independent information that is useful for rational subunit vaccine development.

At the first level of inspection one can compare the genomes of the *Chlamydia* strains used in each model. The *Chlamydophila caviae* genome has been sequenced. There is good synteny (gene order alignment) between *C. trachomatis* serovar D except at the origin of replication and a region of genetic divergence known as the plasticity zone (PZ) or replication termination region [24]. *C. trachomatis* serovar D has 894 open reading frames (genes), 808 of which are shared with *C. cavaie*. It is likely that *C. trachomatis-C. caviae* homologs for these 808 genes have the same role in the host-pathogen relationship, and, from the T cell epitope perspective, likely have similar exposure to the host cell antigen processing machinery.

C. muridarum is even more closely related to *C. trachomatis* serovar D [25]. There are gene-for-gene homologs in identical gene order with the only major differences occurring in the PZ. 810 open reading frames are shared between *C. muridarum* and *C. trachomatis* serovar D, and they likely have similar exposure to the host cell antigen processing machinery. The PZ of human urogenital strains, including serovar D, contains a tryptophan operon capable of synthesizing tryptophan using indole as the precursor (as does *C. caviae*), while the *C. muridarum* PZ has cytotoxin genes with homology to *Yersinia YopT* (as does *C. caviae*). In vitro and in vivo studies support the hypothesis that differences in PZ genes between *C. trachomatis* and *C. mu-*

ridarum are adaptations to species-specific innate defense mechanisms triggered by IFN-γ [26].

Human reproductive tract epithelial cells have IFN-γ-inducible expression of indoleamine-2,3-deoxygenase (IDO), an innate defense that acts against intracellular parasites by depleting intracellular pools of tryptophan, an essential amino acid for many microbial pathogens. Murine reproductive tract epithelial cell lines do not express IDO, with or without IFN-γ treatment. Human *C. trachomatis* urogenital serovars replicating in human epithelial cells can be rescued from IFN-γ-mediated replication inhibition by addition of indole to the medium, presumably by synthesizing tryptophan from the indole precursor. Conversely, *C. muridarum* replication in human epithelial cells is inhibited by IFN-γ and is not rescued by addition of indole to the media, presumably because *C. muridarum* cannot bypass IDO depletion of intracellular tryptophan without a tryptophan synthetase operon [26]. Many laboratory workers have been infected by human *C. trachomatis* strains while no laboratory worker has ever been reported to be infected by *C. muridarum* [27]. It is likely that *C. muridarum* lacks species-specific adaptations, including a tryptophan synthetase operon necessary to replicate in humans.

C. muridarum has three cytotoxin genes in its PZ [26]. In vitro and in vivo data support the hypothesis that the murine cytotoxin genes are a species-specific adaptation to an innate defense mechanism unique to mice mediated by IFN-γ-inducible p47 GTPases. Human *C. trachomatis* urogenital serovars do not have cytotoxin genes, likely because their human host does not have IFN-γ-inducible p47 GTPases. *C. muridarum* replicating in mouse epithelial cell lines is largely indifferent to effects of IFN-γ, presumably because murine epithelial cells do not express IDO and *C. muridarum* cytotoxin genes, by homology to *Yersinia YopT*, likely inactivate IFN-γ-induced murine p47 GTPases. p47 GTPases appear to function as an innate defense against intracellular parasites by disrupting intracellular vesicular trafficking, thereby starving parasitophorous vacuoles of nutrients, including sphingomyelin [26], an essential lipid for *Chlamydia* replication, and/or directing early inclusions to lysosomes [28]. Human *C. trachomatis* strains are unable to replicate in mouse epithelial cells treated with IFN-γ, presumably because they have no answer for the mouse-specific p47 GTPase defense system. Human *C. trachomatis* strains have a very limited replication capability in the murine genital tract compared to *C. muridarum* [29, 30], and are likely overly sensitive to innate defenses induced by IFN-γ, potentially lowering the bar for defining protective host defense in that model system.

In summary, human *C. trachomatis* urogenital strains and rodent *C. muridarum* have evolved different mechanisms for evading species-specific innate defenses induced by IFN-γ. As long as they are in their natural host species, replication of human and murine *Chlamydia* strains is largely indifferent to first level innate defenses induced by IFN-γ. For the purposes of studying adaptive immunity, differences in innate IFN-γ biology are probably not important as long as the *Chlamydia* species used is in its natural host species. Innate host defenses do not resolve *Chlamydia* infections but are critically important for their contributions to immunopathology (addressed at the end of this chapter). Chlamydial genital tract infections are ultimately cleared by an adaptive immune response.

The Adaptive Immune Response and Protective Host Immunity

Early seminal work in the field showed that T cells were critical for clearance of chlamydial genital tract infections [31]. Mice deficient in T cells were unable to clear infections [32]. Interrupting genital tract infections in mice with antibiotic therapy before the tenth day of infection had detrimental effects on the development of protective T cell-mediated immunity [33], potentially explaining somewhat counterproductive antibiotic-based public health strategies as interrupted development of protective T cell-mediated immunity in antibiotic-treated individuals, with a cumulative negative effect on herd immunity [34, 35]. Additional work showed that T cells are sufficient to clear primary genital tract infections, but that there is a role for antibody in clearing secondary challenges after resolution of primary infections [36], and a role for antibody in vaccine-induced immunity [37, 38]. With that general introduction, we will attempt to synthesize a working paradigm for host immunity against genital tract chlamydial infections and point out areas where we still lack knowledge.

The T Cell Response

Data from mouse models strongly support a dominant role for CD4 T cells in protective immunity [39, 40]. Early hypotheses in the field looked toward a role for CD8 T lymphocytes in immune-mediated clearance because *Chlamydia* species are intracellular pathogens [41, 42]. However, a critical role for CD8 T cells in clearance of *Chlamydia* from the genital tract was set aside by experiments utilizing β_2 microglobulin-deficient mice [40]. β_2 microglobulin is a critical component of MHC class I heterodimers (human equivalents are HLA-A and HLA-B) that present foreign peptides to CD8 T cells. Despite a paucity of CD8 T cells and MHC class I molecules, β_2 microglobulin-deficient mice cleared *C. muridarum* genital tract infections with kinetics similar to that of wild-type controls. More recently, *Chlamydia*-specific CD8 T cells have fallen further from grace as they appear to contribute to infertility in the *C. muridarum* mouse model [43]. Mice sufficient in CD8 T cells and B cells have lower fertility rates (greater infertility) than mice sufficient in CD4 T cells and B cells after clearing primary and secondary *C. muridarum* genital tract infections. By extrapolation, vaccine strategies focused on generating MHC class I-restricted CD8 T cell responses may have limited efficacy and could promote detrimental immunopathogy, e.g. infertility.

The most precise statement of protective immunity in the mouse model is that it is critically dependent on MHC class II [40]. MHC class II heterodimers present foreign peptides to CD4 T cells. Mice deficient in MHC class II are unable to clear primary *C. muridarum* genital tract infections. These data and supporting CD4 T cell depletion studies are broadly interpreted as showing a dominant role for CD4 T cells, and no significant role for CD8 T cells in the clearance of infection. This generalization risks being overly broad and may obscure consideration of important CD8 immunobiology. The relevant caveats are that CD8 T cell responses are frequently dependent on CD4 T cell responses during primary infections, and that CD4-deficient mice are able to clear *C. muridarum* genital tract infections with a relatively modest 10-day delay compared to wild-type control mice [40]. *Chlamydia*-specific CD8 T cells in humans are predominantly HLA-A and HLA-B unrestricted [44, 45], i.e. very unusual. In mice, MHC class II-restricted CD8 T cells comprise roughly 10% of 'normal' cellular immune responses [46]. Our understanding of *Chlamydia*-specific CD8 T cell immunobiology is incomplete, and it may be important for understanding host defense, especially immunopathogenesis attributable to the CD8 T cell subset.

CD4 T cells play the dominant role in protective immunity in the mouse model. The critical issues for understanding protective host immunity are: (1) which CD4 T cell subset(s) mediate protection and (2) by what mechanism? A useful parameter for categorizing protective immunity is the immunobiology of IFN-γ. IFN-γ has already come up in the context of its role in innate host defenses (IDO and p47 GTPases). IFN-γ is also an integral component of adaptive immunity. It has important effects on antigen presentation including the transition to immunoproteosomes that process foreign proteins into antigenic peptides (T cell epitopes), and upregulation of MHC class I, MHC class II and ICAM-1 on professional (dendritic cells, macrophages, B cells) and semiprofessional antigen-presenting cells (epithelial cells). Epithelial cells express very little MHC class II unless exposed to IFN-γ. Upregulation of MHC class II is likely critical in host defense against *C. trachomatis* replicating in epithelial cells lining the reproductive tract because CD4 T cells utilize MHC class II to 'see' infected epithelial targets. Mice deficient in MHC class II cannot clear *Chlamydia*. A correlation between IFN-γ-induced MHC class II and CD4 T cell recognition of *C. muridarum*-infected epithelial cells has been demonstrated in vitro [47]. IFN-γ also upregulates expression of epithelial-inducible nitric oxide synthetase (iNOS) that generates nitric oxide, the effector molecule for one of the two known CD4 T cell-mediated mechanisms for controlling *Chlamydia* replication in epithelial cells.

IFN-γ-Dependent Cellular Immunity (iNOS)

T cell surveillance of mucosal epithelium is a unique facet of adaptive cellular immunity, about which we have only a limited understanding. Because replication *of C. trachomatis* urogenital serovars D-K is largely limited to reproductive tract epithelium, it is reasonable to presume that protective CD4 T cell responses must terminate *C. trachomatis* replication in epithelial cells. A universal feature of adaptive T cell immunity is the ability of T cells to 'see' infected cells presenting microbial peptides bound to antigen presentation molecules on their cell surface; therefore, CD4 T cells likely need to interact physically with infected epithelial cells to mediate protective immunity. Consistent with general features of adaptive cellular immunity, the first CD4 T cell-mediated mechanism for terminating *Chlamydia* replication in epithelial cells requires physical interaction between T cells and infected epithelial cells.

CD4 T cells can terminate *Chlamydia* replication by upregulating expression of epithelial-inducible iNOS to generate *Chlamydiacidal* levels of nitric oxide, a chemical antiseptic analogous to hydrogen peroxide. This mechanism requires IFN-γ, and physical contact between CD4 T cells and infected epithelial cells via LFA-1 on the T cell interacting with ICAM-1 on the epithelial cell [48]. IFN-γ alone induces iNOS transcription in epithelial cells, but the physical interaction is required to boost nitric oxide levels to sterilizing levels.

A CD4 protective mechanism mediated by IFN-γ/iNOS/nitric oxide was a satisfying mechanism for controlling an intracellular pathogen such as *C. trachomatis*. However, as is common to biologic systems, the reality of protective immunity is more complex than the initial glimpse at its mechanism. Mice deficient in iNOS were not compromised in clearance of *C. muridarum* genital tract infections [49, 50], and IFN-γ-knockout mice cleared 99.9% of *C. muridarum* from the genital tract with near normal kinetics [31, 51]. This was disconcerting, as were subsequent experiments showing that mechanisms for killing/lysing infected epithelial cells via perforin and FasL were also dispensable for clearing *C. muridarum* from the genital tract [52]. If induction of nitric oxide production and physical killing of infected epithelial cells were not critical, and antibodies were not critical, then there was no known host defense mechanism for understanding resolution of *C. muridarum* genital tract infections. However, critical experiments showed that iNOS was important for sterilizing immunity [53]. Viable *C. muridarum* could be recovered from the genital tracts of iNOS-deficient but not wild-type mice that previously self-cleared genital tract infections when they were treated with cyclophosphamide, a cytoxic drug that depletes lymphocytes and neutrophils more efficiently than monocyte/macrophages.

The IFN-γ and iNOS knockout mouse data showed that sterilizing immunity was dependent on IFN-γ and iNOS, but also that there were IFN-γ- and iNOS-independent mechanisms for clearing *C. muridarum* from the genital tract. It was perplexing that neither iNOS nor T cell-mediated lysis of infected epithelial cells were critical for controlling genital tract infections as knockout mice singly deficient in either function could still clear infection. The existing data could be readily explained if there were two or more redundant CD4 T cell mechanisms for terminating *Chlamydia* replication in epithelial cells.

Evidence for an iNOS and IFN-γ-independent CD4 T cell mechanism came from in vitro studies utilizing *Chlamydia*-specific CD4 T cell clones [54]. In a panel of *Chlamydia*-specific CD4 T cell clones derived from mice that self-cleared *C. muridarum* genital tract infections, it was noted that some clones were better than others at controlling *C. muridarum* replication in epithelial cells. The best clones were able to terminate *C. muridarum* replication in the absence of exogenous IFN-γ and in the presence of inhibitors of iNOS. Blocking the ability of this potent subset of CD4 T cell clones required both inhibition of iNOS and inhibition of T cell degranulation. This was evidence for a second mechanism that was not dependent on nitric oxide production. Because these same T cell clones could not recognize infected epithelial cells until 15–18 h postinfection, and could not physically lyse them until >30 h postinfection (*C. muridarum* replication in epithelial cells completed; noninfectious reticulate body → infectious EB transition was over), it was unlikely that physical destruction of the epithelial 'Chlamydia incubator' was the relevant mechanism for terminating infection. The existing data suggested that the iNOS-independent pathway (degranulation dependent) involved injection of a preformed T cell *Chlamydia* microbicide into the epithelial cytosol that directly attacked EBs.

The major T cell granule microbicide in humans is granulysin. However, mice do not have a granulysin homolog, implying existence of an additional T cell microbicide active against *Chlamydia*. Microarray experiments comparing expression of the most potent CD4 T cell clones to less effective CD4 T cell clones identified a small cysteine-rich protein known as *Plac8* (also called onzin) as a candidate T cell granule *Chlamydia* microbicide [55]. Mice deficient in *Plac8* are more susceptible to *Klebsiella* peritonitis [56], implying at least an indirect antibacterial function. The *Chlamydia*-specific CD4 microarray data was followed by infectious challenge of *Plac8*-deficient mice that revealed a compromised ability to clear *C. muridarum* genital tract infections. *Plac8* knockout mice have a ~20-day delay in clearance of *C. muridarum* compared to wild-type controls. Continuous treatment of *Plac8* knockout mice with the iNOS inhibitor N-monomethyl-L-arginine rendered *Plac8* knockout, but not wild-type mice, nearly incapable of clearing a genital tract infection over 8 weeks. That experiment demonstrated redundant mechanisms for clearing *C. muridarum*; one dependent on iNOS, the other dependent on *Plac8*. Mice deficient in either *Plac8* or iNOS could clear a *C. muridarum* genital tract infection, but dual-deficient mice, genetically deficient in *Plac8* and pharmacologically deficient in nitric oxide production, were severely compromised in their ability to clear infection [55].

Plac8 is a 12.4-kd protein that localizes to neutrophil granules and is expressed by a subset of T cells. Confusingly it does not have a conventional signal peptide to put it into vesicular trafficking pathways necessary for delivery to granules. However, its copurification with granules and absence from cytosolic cell fractions argues that it is in the granule, and likely has an unconventional signal peptide. Details about *Plac8*s role as either the facilitator or effector molecule for the iNOS-independent mechanism for terminating *C. muridarum* replication in epithelial cells remains to be determined. Until that *Plac8* biology is clarified it is unclear whether *Plac8* directly kills EBs or facilitates an unknown effector molecule that does.

Cytokine Polarization

For the past 2 decades, the working paradigm for T cell-mediated host defense and immunopathology has focused on cytokine polarization patterns of CD4 and, to a lesser extent, CD8 T cells. The first major CD4 subdivision described was Th1 versus Th2 [57]. Th1 CD4 T cells secrete IFN-γ with or without IL-2, while Th2 T cells secrete IL-4/IL-13 without IFN-γ or IL-2. T cell polarization reflected antagonistic effects of IFN-γ and IL-4 on naïve T cell differentiation. IFN-γ blocked Th2 development dependent on GATA-3, and IL-4 blocked Th1 development dependent on T-bet. In broad strokes, Th1 T cells are specialized to defend against intracellular microbial pathogens by direct action and by facilitating expansion of CD8 cytotoxic T lymphocytes; Th2 T cells are specialized to deal with extracellular pathogens, especially parasites, by facilitating B cell expansion, Ig production and recruitment of eosinophils. Consistent with these general principles, protective responses against *Chlamydia* are Th1 while Th2 responses are ineffective or worsen the infection [58, 59]. The poor performance of Th2 cells in clearing infection could be understood as an inability to utilize the IFN-γ/iNOS-dependent protection mechanism. It is noteworthy that not all *Chlamydia*-specific Th1 T cells are protective in vitro [60] or in vivo [61]. The latter may reflect specificity for nonprotective T cell epitopes, poor homing, lack of TNF-α, or potentially the lack of the *Plac8* mechanism for controlling infection.

In recent years there has been an expansion in helper T cell subsets to include Th3 (mucosal tolerance), Treg (mucosal and peripheral tolerance), Th17 (neutrophil recruitment), Th21 (follicular T cells) and Th22 (epithelial defense activation). In addition, there is an important category of Th1 T cells that deserve their own subset, but are currently referred to as multifunctional Th1 T cells [62]. Activated multifunctional Th1 cells secrete IFN-γ, TNF-α and IL-2, and correlate with protective immunity in vaccine studies in the *C. muridarum* mouse model [63, 64]. That finding is consistent with the finding that TNF-α receptor-deficient mice are less efficient in clearing *C. muridarum* infections [31]. The stature of TNF-α is further enhanced by the finding that Th1 cells that produce only IFN-γ upon activation do not appear to mediate protection in the *C. muridarum* mouse vaccine model [63]. TNF-α may be a mechanism-crossover cytokine. In the presence of IFN-γ, TNF-α boosts induction of iNOS expression via NFkB binding sites in the iNOS promoter [65], and induces expression of epithelial ICAM-1, facilitating epithelial nitric oxide production via T cell-epithelial cell interaction [48]. Multifunctional CD4 T cells also have more robust degranulation [66] that may have a bearing on *Plac8*-dependent cellular immunity.

The understanding of Th17 and Th22 immunobiology is in early stages, and their roles in *Chlamydia* biology remain to be determined. This is a major semantic issue in the current literature. It is unclear whether making IL-17 upon activation is the equivalent of being a Th17 cell. For the most part, Th17 T cells are an in vitro CD4 T cell subset generated by activating naïve CD4 T cells in the presence of TGF-β and IL-6, or IL-21 ± IL-23 while neutralizing IFN-γ. This combination generates RORγt-positive T cells that produce IL-17 and no IFN-γ upon activation. It is now clear in vivo that many IL-17-positive T cells are also IFN-γ positive [63]. Polarizing naïve *Chlamydia*-specific CD4 transgenic T cells to a Th17 phenotype was readily accomplished in vitro; however, when those T cells were adoptively transferred and mice infected with *C. trachomatis* serovar L2, the recovered transgenic T cells were IFN-γ positive, ±TNF-α, with a modest frequency of IL-17 [59]. It is likely that multifunctional CD4 T cells producing IFN-γ and IL-17 is the cytokine polarization event more relevant to *Chlamydia* immunobiology.

T cell production of IL-17, whichever subset produces it, is an emerging cytokine in *Chlamydia* immunobiology. The role of IL-17 is to protect against bacterial infections, generally extracellular bacteria, by recruiting and activating neutrophils. IL-17 also has a major role in immunopathology, most prominently demonstrated for autoimmune rheumatoid arthritis. Recruitment of and activation of neutrophils has potential for destruction of delicate reproductive tract architecture via release of metalloproteases and elastases. Existing data from the mouse model suggests that IL-17 has a modest role in controlling *Chlamydia* replication in the lung [67]. One study in the *C. muridarum* mouse model failed to show any effect of neutralizing IL-17 antibody therapy on bacterial loads or pathology during genital tract infections [68]. These studies may be somewhat biased against a positive result because IL-17 exists as IL-17a/a, IL-17f/f, and IL-17a/f heterodimers, while the available antibody reagent for neutralization was IL-17a specific. IL-22 is an interesting cytokine because it activates epithelial cell defense mechanisms including expression of defensins; however, there are currently no *Chlamydia*-specific data addressing this cytokine or T cell subset other than documentation of their presence in cervical CD4 T cells of *C. trachomatis*-infected women [69].

In summary, CD4 T cell cytokines have important roles in *Chlamydia* immunobiology. The best evidence for protective immunity suggests that multifunctional Th1 cells mediate protective immunity, possibly by augmenting iNOS-dependent and degranulation-dependent immune mechanisms. Not surprisingly, Th2 T cells are ineffectual and predispose to detrimental immunopathology, likely because they cannot utilize the iNOS-mediated clearance mechanism. Surprisingly, Th1 cells producing only IFN-γ on activation appear to be ineffective for protective immunity, highlighting the importance of multifunctional Th1 cells and TNF-α. The newcomer on the CD4 T cell subset block, Th17, or at least T cells that make IL-17, have an unclear role in *Chlamydia* protection and immunopathogenesis. With the discovery of a *Plac8*-dependent clearance mechanism, the role of CD4$_{Plac8}$ T cells in protective immunity is an important topic for future research.

Antibody-Mediated Immunity

Antibodies are not critical for clearance of primary *Chlamydia* genital tract infections in animal models. B cell-deficient mice clear primary infections with normal kinetics [70]. There is, however, a role for B cells and antibody in clearing secondary infections (rechallenge) [36]. Interestingly, the specificity of the antibody seems to be of limited importance. Anti-MOMP, anti-LPS and antiserum from immune mice are all capable of mediating this mechanism. Anti-LPS antibody has no potential to neutralize EBs. In addition, passive transfer of antibody prior to primary infection does not confer any protection to the recipient mice, arguing that antibodies probably do not directly mediate the effect via complement or other innate mechanism (e.g. ADCC). Indirect mechanisms related to enhanced antigen presentation are possibilities. Professional APC bearing antigen-specific surface Ig are 1,000 times more efficient at presenting antigen [71] (i.e. can present antigens present at very low concentrations potentially accelerating an adaptive immune response). A role for Fc receptors in anti-*Chlamydia* secondary responses has been previously demonstrated [72]. Confusingly, antibody depletion of CD4 or CD8, or both CD4 and CD8, after clearance of the primary infection has no effect on this Ig-dependent secondary clearance mechanism [73], begging the question of which effector cell type mediates this mechanism. The antibody dependent secondary clearance mechanism is one of the major remaining mysteries of protective host immunity.

Lack of a critical role for antibodies in clearing primary infections should not be interpreted as meaning that anti-*Chlamydia* antibodies are unimportant. Two recent studies, one combining inactivated EB with an intracellular nonelementary body *Chlamydia* protein and a second study vaccinating B cell-sufficient and deficient mice with native MOMP, have shown improved protection with vaccine strategies that generate anti-*Chlamydia* antibodies [37, 38].

Summary of Adaptive Immunity

In summary, there are three major adaptive immunity mechanisms for clearing *Chlamydia* genital tract infections in the mouse model; two CD4 T cell mechanisms and one antibody-dependent mechanism. The originally described CD4 T cell mechanism is iNOS and IFN-γ dependent, while the second CD4 T cell mechanism

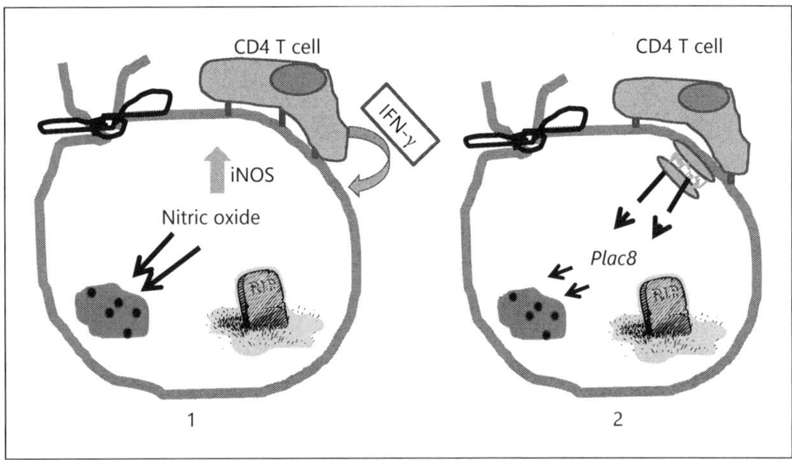

Fig. 1. Toxic bag paradigm: CD4 T cell mechanisms for clearance of *C. muridarum* from the genital tract. 1 = IFN-γ and iNOS dependent; 2 = *Plac8* dependent. Sterilizing immunity requires both 1 and 2.

is *Plac8* dependent (fig. 1). These CD4 T cell mechanisms are potent and singly sufficient (i.e. redundant) for clearing primary genital tract infections; however, sterilizing immunity appears to require both iNOS and *Plac8*. Interestingly, neither iNOS-dependent nor *Plac8*-dependent mechanisms require cytolysis. Instead, both mechanisms neutralize *Chlamydia* trapped within an intact epithelial cell, a 'toxic bag' model of sterilizing immunity. In fact, premature cytolysis would likely be detrimental to both mechanisms. iNOS expression has been demonstrated in epithelial cells lining the human reproductive tract [74], and murine *Plac8* has a highly conserved human homolog [56]. There are no reasons a priori to dismiss iNOS and *Plac8* as the relevant protective mechanisms in humans.

The third adaptive immunity mechanism for clearing *C. muridarum* genital tract infections requires an antibody response and preexisting cellular immunity developed during clearance of a primary infection. Important details of this immunoglobulin-based mechanism remain to be determined.

Innate Immune Response and Immunopathology

The innate immune response is not responsible for resolution of *Chlamydia* genital tract infections as evidenced by the requirement for T lymphocytes. Innate responses are likely responsible for a 2–3 log decrease in *C. muridarum* shedding during the first 10 days of infection, the timeframe in which antibiotic treatment interferes with development of a protective secondary T cell response. This window corresponds to peak levels of IFN-γ and TNF-α in genital tract secretions, which reach a maximum on day ~4 then taper to low levels by day 14 [68]. This early innate blast of IFN-γ and TNF-α likely accounts for poor replication capacity of human urogenital serovars in the mouse [30, 31], and the early 2 log decrease in *C. muridarum* shedding in wild-type mice. IFN-γ and TNF-α synergize to induce iNOS transcription and nitric oxide production. Both human and mouse *Chlamydia* strains are susceptible to high levels of nitric oxide [48, 75]. In mice the innate anti-*Chlamydia* mechanisms relevant to human strains likely include p47 GTPases and nitric oxide, and for *C. muridarum* exclusively nitric oxide. Mice deficient in MyD88, signaling molecule for TLR2 (also TLR4, 5, 7–9), have delayed clearance of *C. muridarum* from the genital tract [76]. MyD88 mice turn out to be deficient in the early innate blast of IFN-γ provided by natural killer cells [77], and also have delayed recruitment of CD4 T cells to the reproductive tract that likely explain the delay in clearance, highlighting the bridge between innate and adaptive immunity [76].

Innate IFN-α/β responses antagonize IFN-γ-mediated protection as type 1 interferon receptor-deficient mice clear infection faster than wild-type controls with less immunopathology [78]. Complementary in vitro data has shown that IFN-β blocks IFN-γ-mediated upregulation of epithelial MHC class II and dampens *Chlamydia*-specific CD4 T cell activation [47]. It is possible that the balance between type I and type II interferon responses within individuals is a contributing factor to clearance and immunopathology. Infected epithelial cells and macrophages are sources of type I interferons via different TLR pathways [79, 80].

TLRs play a critical role in immunopathology in the mouse model. While TLRs differ between mice (TLRs 1–9 and 11–13) and humans (TLRs 1–10), TLR2, the TLR critical for immunopathology, is conserved in sequence (79% conserved; 71% identical) and function (ligand recognition of bacterial lipids and lipopeptides) between mice and humans. Mice deficient in TLR2 have lower levels of TNF-α and CXCL2 (MIP-2; chemokine for recruiting neutrophils) in genital tract secretions, and less immunopathology than control mice, without any difference in clearance kinetics [81]. Complementary in vitro data with oviduct epithelial cells identified TLR2/MyD88 as the pathway responsible for infected epithelial production of inflammatory cytokines including IL-6 and GM-CSF [82]. Very interesting observations have been made using a plasmid-deficient *C. muridarum* strain that fails to activate TLR2. Infection of mice with plasmid-deficient *C. muridarum* generated protection against immunopathology on rechallenge with wild-type *C. muridarum*, but surprisingly protection from rechallenge immunopathology was not based on rapid clearance of the secondary infection [83]. These results highlight the complexities involved for those interested in rational vaccine development.

References

1 Agrawal T, Vats V, Salhan S, Mittal A: Mucosal and peripheral immune responses to chlamydial heat shock proteins in women infected with *Chlamydia trachomatis*. Clin Exp Immunol 2007;148:461–468.

2 Pate MS, Hedges SR, Sibley DA, Russell MW, Hook EW 3rd, Mestecky J: Urethral cytokine and immune responses in *Chlamydia trachomatis*-infected males. Infect Immun 2001;69:7178–7181.

3 Wang C, Tang J, Crowley-Nowick PA, Wilson CM, Kaslow RA, Geisler WM: Interleukin (IL)-2 and IL-12 responses to *Chlamydia trachomatis* infection in adolescents. Clin Exp Immunol 2005;142:548–554.

4 Geisler WM, Yu S, Hook EW 3rd: Chlamydial and gonococcal infection in men without polymorphonuclear leukocytes on gram stain: implications for diagnostic approach and management. Sex Transm Dis 2005;32:630–634.

5 Mittal A, Rastogi S, Reddy BS, Verma S, Salhan S, Gupta E: Enhanced immunocompetent cells in chlamydial cervicitis. J Reprod Med 2004;49:671–677.

6 Ghaem-Maghami S, Ratti G, Ghaem-Maghami M, Comanducci M, Hay PE, Bailey RL, Mabey DC, Whittle HC, Ward ME, Lewis DJ: Mucosal and systemic immune responses to plasmid protein pgp3 in patients with genital and ocular *Chlamydia trachomatis* infection. Clin Exp Immunol 2003;132:436–442.

7 Mittal A, Kapur S, Gupta S: Host immune response in chlamydial cervicitis. Br J Biomed Sci 1996;53:214–220.

8 Cohen CR, Koochesfahani KM, Meier AS, Shen C, Karunakaran K, Ondondo B, Kinyari T, Mugo NR, Nguti R, Brunham RC: Immunoepidemiologic profile of *Chlamydia trachomatis* infection: importance of heat-shock protein 60 and interferon-γ. J Infect Dis 2005;192:591–599.

9 Debattista J, Timms P, Allan J: Reduced levels of gamma-interferon secretion in response to chlamydial 60 kDa heat shock protein amongst women with pelvic inflammatory disease and a history of repeated *Chlamydia trachomatis* infections. Immunol Lett 2002;81:205–210.

10 Hosenfeld CB, Workowski KA, Berman S, Zaidi A, Dyson J, Mosure D, Bolan G, Bauer HM: Repeat infection with Chlamydia and gonorrhea among females: a systematic review of the literature. Sex Transm Dis 2009;36:478–489.

11 Dunne EF, Chapin JB, Rietmeijer CA, Kent CK, Ellen JM, Gaydos CA, Willard NJ, Kohn R, Lloyd L, Thomas S, Birkjukow N, Chung S, Klausner J, Schillinger JA, Markowitz LE: Rate and predictors of repeat *Chlamydia trachomatis* infection among men. Sex Transm Dis 2008;35:S40–S44.

12 Katz BP, Batteiger BE, Jones RB: Effect of prior sexually transmitted disease on the isolation of *Chlamydia trachomatis*. Sex Transm Dis 1987;14:160–164.

13 Brunham RC, Kimani J, Bwayo J, Maitha G, Maclean I, Yang C, Shen C, Roman S, Nagelkerke NJ, Cheang M, Plummer FA: The epidemiology of *Chlamydia trachomatis* within a sexually transmitted diseases core group. J Infect Dis 1996;173:950–956.

14 Geisler WM: Duration of untreated, uncomplicated *Chlamydia trachomatis* genital infection and factors associated with chlamydia resolution: a review of human studies. J Infect Dis 2010;201(suppl 2):S104–S113.

15 Wang C, Tang J, Geisler WM, Crowley-Nowick PA, Wilson CM, Kaslow RA: Human leukocyte antigen and cytokine gene variants as predictors of recurrent *Chlamydia trachomatis* infection in high-risk adolescents. J Infect Dis 2005;191:1084–1092.

16 Cohen CR, Gichui J, Rukaria R, Sinei SS, Gaur LK, Brunham RC: Immunogenetic correlates for *Chlamydia trachomatis*-associated tubal infertility. Obstet Gynecol 2003;101:438–444.

17 Kinnunen AH, Surcel HM, Lehtinen M, Karhukorpi J, Tiitinen A, Halttunen M, Bloigu A, Morrison RP, Karttunen R, Paavonen J: HLA DQ alleles and interleukin-10 polymorphism associated with *Chlamydia trachomatis*-related tubal factor infertility: a case-control study. Hum Reprod 2002;17:2073–2078.

18 Cohen CR, Sinei SS, Bukusi EA, Bwayo JJ, Holmes KK, Brunham RC: Human leukocyte antigen class II DQ alleles associated with *Chlamydia trachomatis* tubal infertility. Obstet Gynecol 2000;95:72–77.

19 Ness RB, Brunham RC, Shen C, Bass DC: Associations among human leukocyte antigen (HLA) class II DQ variants, bacterial sexually transmitted diseases, endometritis, and fertility among women with clinical pelvic inflammatory disease. Sex Transm Dis 2004;31:301–304.

20 Brunham RC, Kuo CC, Cles L, Holmes KK: Correlation of host immune response with quantitative recovery of *Chlamydia trachomatis* from the human endocervix. Infect Immun 1983;39:1491–1494.

21 Cunningham DS: Immune response characteristics in women with chlamydial genital tract infection. Gynecol Obstet Invest 1995;39:54–59.

22 Rank RG, Sanders MM: Pathogenesis of endometritis and salpingitis in a guinea pig model of chlamydial genital infection. Am J Pathol 1992;140:927–936.

23 Rank RG, Bowlin AK, Reed RL, Darville T: Characterization of chlamydial genital infection resulting from sexual transmission from male to female guinea pigs and determination of infectious dose. Infect Immun 2003;71:6148–6154.

24 Read TD, Myers GS, Brunham RC, Nelson WC, Paulsen IT, Heidelberg J, Holtzapple E, Khouri H, Federova NB, Carty HA, Umayam LA, Haft DH, Peterson J, Beanan MJ, White O, Salzberg SL, Hsia RC, McClarty G, Rank RG, Bavoil PM, Fraser CM: Genome sequence of *Chlamydophila caviae* (*Chlamydia psittaci* GPIC): examining the role of niche-specific genes in the evolution of the Chlamydiaceae. Nucleic Acids Res 2003;31:2134–2147.

25 Read TD, Brunham RC, Shen C, Gill SR, Heidelberg JF, White O, Hickey EK, Peterson J, Utterback T, Berry K, Bass S, Linher K, Weidman J, Khouri H, Craven B, Bowman C, Dodson R, Gwinn M, Nelson W, DeBoy R, Kolonay J, McClarty G, Salzberg SL, Eisen J, Fraser CM: Genome sequences of *Chlamydia trachomatis* MoPn and *Chlamydia pneumoniae* AR39. Nucleic Acids Res 2000;28:1397–1406.

26 Nelson DE, Virok DP, Wood H, Roshick C, Johnson RM, Whitmire WM, Crane DD, Steele-Mortimer O, Kari L, McClarty G, Caldwell HD: Chlamydial IFN-γ immune evasion is linked to host infection tropism. Proc Natl Acad Sci USA 2005;102:10658–10663.

27 Miller CD, Songer JR, Sullivan JF: A twenty-five year review of laboratory-acquired human infections at the National Animal Disease Center. Am Ind Hyg Assoc J 1987;48:271–275.

28 Al-Zeer MA, Al-Younes HM, Braun PR, Zerrahn J, Meyer TF: IFN-γ-inducible Irga6 mediates host resistance against *Chlamydia trachomatis* via autophagy. PLoS One 2009;4:e4588.

29 Morrison SG, Farris CM, Sturdevant GL, Whitmire WM, Morrison RP: Murine *Chlamydia trachomatis* genital infection is unaltered by depletion of CD4+ T cells and diminished adaptive immunity. J Infect Dis 2011;203:1120–1128.

30 Perry LL, Feilzer K, Caldwell HD: Immunity to *Chlamydia trachomatis* is mediated by T helper 1 cells through IFN-γ-dependent and -independent pathways. J Immunol 1997;158:3344–3352.

31 Rank RG, Barron AL: Effect of antithymocyte serum on the course of chlamydial genital infection in female guinea pigs. Infect Immun 1983;41:876–879.

32 Rank RG, Soderberg LS, Barron AL: Chronic chlamydial genital infection in congenitally athymic nude mice. Infect Immun 1985;48:847–849.

33 Su H, Morrison R, Messer R, Whitmire W, Hughes S, Caldwell HD: The effect of doxycycline treatment on the development of protective immunity in a murine model of chlamydial genital infection. J Infect Dis 1999;180:1252–1258.

34 Brunham RC, Pourbohloul B, Mak S, White R, Rekart ML: The unexpected impact of a *Chlamydia trachomatis* infection control program on susceptibility to reinfection. J Infect Dis 2005;192:1836–1844.

35 Brunham RC, Rekart ML: The arrested immunity hypothesis and the epidemiology of chlamydia control. Sex Transm Dis 2008;35:53–54.

36 Morrison SG, Morrison RP: A predominant role for antibody in acquired immunity to chlamydial genital tract reinfection. J Immunol 2005;175:7536–7542.

37 Farris CM, Morrison SG, Morrison RP: CD4+ T cells and antibody are required for optimal major outer membrane protein vaccine-induced immunity to *Chlamydia muridarum* genital infection. Infect Immun 2010;78:4374–4383.

38 Li W, Murthy AK, Guentzel MN, Chambers JP, Forsthuber TG, Seshu J, Zhong G, Arulanandam BP: Immunization with a combination of integral chlamydial antigens and a defined secreted protein induces robust immunity against genital chlamydial challenge. Infect Immun 2010;78:3942–3949.

39 Morrison RP, Caldwell HD: Immunity to murine chlamydial genital infection. Infect Immun 2002;70: 2741–2751.

40 Morrison RP, Feilzer K, Tumas DB: Gene knockout mice establish a primary protective role for major histocompatibility complex class II-restricted responses in *Chlamydia trachomatis* genital tract infection. Infect Immun 1995;63:4661–4668.

41 Starnbach MN, Bevan MJ, Lampe MF: Protective cytotoxic T lymphocytes are induced during murine infection with *Chlamydia trachomatis*. J Immunol 1994;153:5183–5189.

42 Igietseme JU, Magee DM, Williams DM, Rank RG: Role for CD8+ T cells in antichlamydial immunity defined by Chlamydia-specific T-lymphocyte clones. Infect Immun 1994;62:5195–5197.

43 Igietseme JU, He Q, Joseph K, Eko FO, Lyn D, Ananaba G, Campbell A, Bandea C, Black CM: Role of T lymphocytes in the pathogenesis of Chlamydia disease. J Infect Dis 2009;200:926–934.

44 Matyszak MK, Gaston JS: *Chlamydia trachomatis*-specific human CD8+ T cells show two patterns of antigen recognition. Infect Immun 2004;72:4357–4367.

45 Gervassi AL, Probst P, Stamm WE, Marrazzo J, Grabstein KH, Alderson MR: Functional characterization of class Ia- and non-class Ia-restricted Chlamydia-reactive CD8+ T cell responses in humans. J Immunol 2003;171:4278–4286.

46 Golding H, Singer A: Specificity, phenotype, and precursor frequency of primary cytolytic T lymphocytes specific for class II major histocompatibility antigens. J Immunol 1985;135:1610–1615.

47 Jayarapu K, Kerr MS, Katschke A, Johnson RM: *Chlamydia muridarum*-specific CD4 T cell clones recognize infected reproductive tract epithelial cells in an interferon-dependent fashion. Infect Immun 2009;77:4469–4479.

48 Igietseme JU, Uriri IM, Hawkins R, Rank RG: Integrin-mediated epithelial-T cell interaction enhances nitric oxide production and increased intracellular inhibition of Chlamydia. J Leukoc Biol 1996;59:656–662.

49 Igietseme JU, Perry LL, Ananaba GA, Uriri IM, Ojior OO, Kumar SN, Caldwell HD: Chlamydial infection in inducible nitric oxide synthase knockout mice. Infect Immun 1998;66:1282–1286.

50 Ramsey KH, Miranpuri GS, Poulsen CE, Marthakis NB, Braune LM, Byrne GI: Inducible nitric oxide synthase does not affect resolution of murine chlamydial genital tract infections or eradication of chlamydiae in primary murine cell culture. Infect Immun 1998;66:835–838.

51 Cotter TW, Ramsey KH, Miranpuri GS, Poulsen CE, Byrne GI: Dissemination of *Chlamydia trachomatis* chronic genital tract infection in gamma interferon gene knockout mice. Infect Immun 1997;65:2145–2152.

52 Perry LL, Feilzer K, Hughes S, Caldwell HD: Clearance of *Chlamydia trachomatis* from the murine genital mucosa does not require perforin-mediated cytolysis or Fas-mediated apoptosis. Infect Immun 1999;67:1379–1385.

53 Ramsey KH, Miranpuri GS, Sigar IM, Ouellette S, Byrne GI: *Chlamydia trachomatis* persistence in the female mouse genital tract: inducible nitric oxide synthase and infection outcome. Infect Immun 2001;69:5131–5137.

54 Jayarapu K, Kerr M, Ofner S, Johnson RM: Chlamydia-specific CD4 T cell clones control *Chlamydia muridarum* replication in epithelial cells by nitric oxide-dependent and -independent mechanisms. J Immunol 2010;185:6911–6920.

55 Johnson RM, Kerr MS, Slaven JE: Plac8-dependent and iNOS-dependent mechanisms clear *Chlamydia muridarum* infections from the genital tract. J Immunol 2012;188:1896–1904.

56 Ledford JG, Kovarova M, Koller BH: Impaired host defense in mice lacking ONZIN. J Immunol 2007;178:5132–5143.

57 Mosmann TR, Cherwinski H, Bond MW, Giedlin MA, Coffman RL: Two types of murine helper T cell clone. I. Definition according to profiles of lymphokine activities and secreted proteins. J Immunol 1986;136:2348–2357.

58 Hawkins RA, Rank RG, Kelly KA: A *Chlamydia trachomatis*-specific Th2 clone does not provide protection against a genital infection and displays reduced trafficking to the infected genital mucosa. Infect Immun 2002;70:5132–5139.

59 Gondek DC, Roan NR, Starnbach MN: T cell responses in the absence of IFN-γ exacerbate uterine infection with *Chlamydia trachomatis*. J Immunol 2009;183:1313–1319.

60 Igietseme JU, Wyrick PB, Goyeau D, Rank RG: An in vitro model for immune control of chlamydial growth in polarized epithelial cells. Infect Immun 1994;62:3528–3535.

61 Igietseme JU, Ramsey KH, Magee DM, Williams DM, Kincy TJ, Rank RG: Resolution of murine chlamydial genital infection by the adoptive transfer of a biovar-specific, Th1 lymphocyte clone. Reg Immunol 1993;5:317–324.

62 Darrah PA, Patel DT, De Luca PM, Lindsay RW, Davey DF, Flynn BJ, Hoff ST, Andersen P, Reed SG, Morris SL, Roederer M, Seder RA: Multifunctional TH1 cells define a correlate of vaccine-mediated protection against Leishmania major. Nat Med 2007;13:843–850.

63 Yu H, Jiang X, Shen C, Karunakaran KP, Jiang J, Rosin NL, Brunham RC: *Chlamydia muridarum* T cell antigens formulated with the adjuvant DDA/TDB induce immunity against infection that correlates with a high frequency of gamma interferon (IFN-gamma)/tumor necrosis factor alpha and IFN-gamma/interleukin-17 double-positive CD4+ T cells. Infect Immun 2010;78:2272–2282.

64 Yu H, Karunakaran KP, Kelly I, Shen C, Jiang X, Foster LJ, Brunham RC: Immunization with live and dead *Chlamydia muridarum* induces different levels of protective immunity in a murine genital tract model: correlation with MHC class II peptide presentation and multifunctional Th1 cells. J Immunol 2011;186:3615–3621.

65 Drapier JC, Wietzerbin J, Hibbs JB Jr: Interferon-gamma and tumor necrosis factor induce the L-arginine-dependent cytotoxic effector mechanism in murine macrophages. Eur J Immunol 1988;18:1587–1592.

66 Kannanganat S, Ibegbu C, Chennareddi L, Robinson HL, Amara RR: Multiple-cytokine-producing antiviral CD4 T cells are functionally superior to single-cytokine-producing cells. J Virol 2007;81:8468–8476.

67 Zhou X, Chen Q, Moore J, Kolls JK, Halperin S, Wang J: Critical role of the interleukin-17/interleukin-17 receptor axis in regulating host susceptibility to respiratory infection with Chlamydia species. Infect Immun 2009;77:5059–5070.

68 Scurlock AM, Frazer LC, Andrews CW Jr, O'Connell CM, Foote IP, Bailey SL, Chandra-Kuntal K, Kolls JK, Darville T: Interleukin-17 contributes to generation of Th1 immunity and neutrophil recruitment during *Chlamydia muridarum* genital tract infection but is not required for macrophage influx or normal resolution of infection. Infect Immun 2011;79:1349–1362.

69 Jha R, Srivastava P, Salhan S, Finckh A, Gabay C, Mittal A, Bas S: Spontaneous secretion of interleukin-17 and -22 by human cervical cells in *Chlamydia trachomatis* infection. Microbes Infect 2011;13:167–178.

70 Su H, Feilzer K, Caldwell HD, Morrison RP: *Chlamydia trachomatis* genital tract infection of antibody-deficient gene knockout mice. Infect Immun 1997;65:1993–1999.

71 Rock KL, Benacerraf B, Abbas AK: Antigen presentation by hapten-specific B lymphocytes. I. Role of surface immunoglobulin receptors. J Exp Med 1984; 160:1102–1113.

72 Moore T, Ananaba GA, Bolier J, Bowers S, Belay T, Eko FO, Igietseme JU: Fc receptor regulation of protective immunity against *Chlamydia trachomatis*. Immunology 2002;105:213–221.

73 Morrison SG, Morrison RP: Resolution of secondary *Chlamydia trachomatis* genital tract infection in immune mice with depletion of both CD4+ and CD8+ T cells. Infect Immun 2001;69:2643–2649.

74 Tschugguel W, Schneeberger C, Unfried G, Czerwenka K, Weninger W, Mildner M, Bishop JR, Huber JC: Induction of inducible nitric oxide synthase expression in human secretory endometrium. Hum Reprod 1998;13:436–444.

75 Igietseme JU, Uriri IM, Chow M, Abe E, Rank RG: Inhibition of intracellular multiplication of human strains of *Chlamydia trachomatis* by nitric oxide. Biochem Biophys Res Commun 1997;232:595–601.

76 Nagarajan UM, Sikes J, Prantner D, Andrews CW Jr, Frazer L, Goodwin A, Snowden JN, Darville T: MyD88 deficiency leads to decreased NK cell gamma interferon production and T cell recruitment during *Chlamydia muridarum* genital tract infection, but a predominant Th1 response and enhanced monocytic inflammation are associated with infection resolution. Infect Immun 2011;79:486–498.

77 Tseng CT, Rank RG: Role of NK cells in early host response to chlamydial genital infection. Infect Immun 1998;66:5867–5875.

78 Nagarajan UM, Prantner D, Sikes JD, Andrews CW Jr, Goodwin AM, Nagarajan S, Darville T: Type I interferon signaling exacerbates *Chlamydia muridarum* genital infection in a murine model. Infect Immun 2008;76:4642–4648.

79 Derbigny WA, Johnson RM, Toomey KS, Ofner S, Jayarapu K: The *Chlamydia muridarum*-induced IFN-β response is TLR3-dependent in murine oviduct epithelial cells. J Immunol 2010;185:6689–6697.

80 Nagarajan UM, Ojcius DM, Stahl L, Rank RG, Darville T: *Chlamydia trachomatis* induces expression of IFN-γ-inducible protein 10 and IFN-β independent of TLR2 and TLR4, but largely dependent on MyD88. J Immunol 2005;175:450–460.

81 Darville T, O'Neill JM, Andrews CW Jr, Nagarajan UM, Stahl L, Ojcius DM: Toll-like receptor-2, but not Toll-like receptor-4, is essential for development of oviduct pathology in chlamydial genital tract infection. J Immunol 2003;171:6187–6197.

82 Derbigny WA, Kerr MS, Johnson RM: Pattern recognition molecules activated by *Chlamydia muridarum* infection of cloned murine oviduct epithelial cell lines. J Immunol 2005;175:6065–6075.

83 O'Connell CM, Ingalls RR, Andrews CW Jr, Scurlock AM, Darville T: Plasmid-deficient *Chlamydia muridarum* fail to induce immune pathology and protect against oviduct disease. J Immunol 2007;179: 4027–4034.

Raymond M. Johnson, MD, PhD
Associate Professor of Medicine, Microbiology and Immunology
Division of Infectious Diseases, Indiana University School of Medicine
635 Barnhill Drive, No. 224, Indianapolis, IN 46202 (USA)
E-Mail raymjohn@iu.edu

Black CM (ed): Chlamydial Infection: A Clinical and Public Health Perspective.
Issues Infect Dis. Basel, Karger, 2013, vol 7, pp 115–130 (DOI: 10.1159/000348762)

Chlamydia Vaccine Development

Joseph U. Igietseme · Carolyn M. Black

National Center for Emerging Zoonotic and Infectious Diseases, Centers for Disease Control and Prevention,
Atlanta, Ga., USA

Abstract

The search for a safe and efficacious human chlamydial vaccine has been ongoing for more than 5
decades. Unfortunately, the dream has yet to be realized. However, much progress has been made
in defining the immunologic requirements of a potentially efficacious vaccine, which involve the
induction of a strong CD4 T cell-driven Th1 response, as well as an accessory antibody response that
is vital for a rapid and robust memory response to reinfections. While a subunit vaccine is currently
preferred to the whole organism, the vaccine antigen(s) may be a single or a multisubunit, provided
it furnishes ample T and B cell epitopes to induce adequate protective immune responses without
immunopathogenic responses. In addition, any subunit vaccine prospect would require a delivery
vehicle and method that can together produce an effective immunomodulation to both boost the
protective immunity and target immune effectors to the mucosal site of infection. Furthermore, a
vaccine that confers broadly specific and long-term protective immunity against both chlamydial
infection and disease is the ultimate goal; however, a vaccine that prevents only the development
of serious complications (e.g. blinding trachoma, pelvic inflammatory disease, ectopic pregnancy,
infertility and pneumonia) could be an acceptable short-term goal.

Need for a *Chlamydia* Vaccine

Members of the major clinically relevant bacterial species of the genus *Chlamydia*
cause ocular, genital and respiratory infections as pathogens that infect only humans
(e.g. *Chlamydia trachomatis* and *C. pneumoniae*), as zoonotic pathogens (e.g. *C. psittaci*) or as veterinary pathogens (e.g. *C. pecorum* and *C. abortus*). However, all *Chlamydia* species have a similar developmental cycle, comprising two prominent morphologically distinct forms, the infectious elementary body (EB) form and an obligate
intracellular, noninfectious and vegetative form called the reticulate body (RB; see
Introduction to this book for details on the developmental cycle). The public health
significance of chlamydial infections is underscored by the huge socioeconomic bur-

den of the ocular, genital and respiratory diseases, as well as the economic losses in the veterinary industry. Human ocular infections by serovars A, B, Ba and C of *C. trachomatis* cause trachoma, the world's most common preventable blinding disease, essentially an epidemic in several developing nations in Africa, South East Asia and the Middle East. An estimated 150 million people are infected worldwide, of which 6 million are visually impaired or irreversibly blinded [1]. Human genital chlamydial infections and the clinical outcomes account for more than 90 of the 500 million annual new sexually transmitted diseases (STDs) worldwide, thus ranking as the most common bacterial cause of STD [2, 3]; the USA alone spends over USD 3 billion annually on an estimated 4 million reported clinical cases of genital chlamydial infections [4, 5]. In addition to self-limiting urethritis in both males and females, cervicitis in women, and epididymitis and proctitis in men, pelvic inflammatory disease and tubal factor infertility are major complications of female genital chlamydial infection, occurring in approximately 40 and 10% of untreated infections, respectively, and constituting an enormous morbidity and socioeconomic burden [6–9]. Infants who are infected during birth by genitally infected mothers may develop conjunctivitis and respiratory disease that progress to pneumonia. A joint disease called Reiter's syndrome is also a complication of genital chlamydial infection. Finally, reports suggesting that genital chlamydial infection may be rising in some populations [5, 10, 11] and could predispose to HIV-related AIDS [11–18] and human papilloma virus-associated cervical dysplasia have heightened these concerns [3] and the urgency to develop preventive measures. Infections caused by *C. pneumoniae* are rampart in the human population, with approximately over 60% of most American, European and Asian societies being exposed. *C. pneumoniae* infections cause mild to sublethal acute respiratory diseases, such as pharyngitis and bronchitis, and are considered to be responsible for over 10% of community-acquired pneumonia [19]. Initial claims of a possible link between *C. pneumoniae* infection, atherosclerosis and some age-related chronic and autoimmune diseases on the basis of correlative data [20–22] have yet to be substantiated clinically and experimentally. Infections by the zoonotic *C. psittaci* produce an assortment of clinical manifestations which, in animals and birds, are psittacosis, hepatitis, mastitis, conjunctivitis, pneumonia, abortions and diarrhea; in humans, it is a psittacosis-like disease that may, in rare cases, become systemic or fatal pneumonia [23]. *C. psittaci* is thus an occupational hazard for workers in the poultry and farming industry and in persons exposed to infected avian species [24]. Finally, *C. pecorum* causes infectious pneumonitis in domestic animals [25, 26] as a veterinary pathogen.

Considering the magnitude and near epidemic state of ocular, genital and respiratory chlamydial infections in some populations, the continued spread in communities worldwide, and the economic stress on the healthcare system, several prevention and control strategies have been proposed and/or executed. These control and prevention measures include mass screening and treatment, mass antibiotic treatment of at-risk populations, health education programs on prevention methods, and the use of an efficacious vaccine as an immunoprophylaxis and preventive. Interestingly, a number of

Table 1. Proposed chlamydial control and prevention measures, advantages and limitations

Chlamydial control and prevention measure	Advantages	Disadvantages
Targeted and/or mass screening and treatment	Treatment of diagnosed cases to: Prevent transmission and spread of infections Prevent evolution of infections to complications/sequelae (pelvic inflammatory disease, infertility, trachoma, etc.)	Population coverage may be infeasible Indiscriminate use of antibiotics may create selection pressure for producing resistant strains Misdiagnosed (false negative) cases that are not treated (due to assay or technical or other errors) may lead to continued spread of infections and diseases Will early treatment cause arrested immunity?
Mass treatment of populations or communities	Indiscriminate mass treatment could: Prevent the transmission and spread of infections Prevent evolution of infections to complications/sequelae (pelvic inflammatory disease, infertility, trachoma, etc.)	Population coverage may be infeasible Indiscriminate use of antibiotics may create selection pressure for emergence of resistant strains Cost in most societies may be unattainable! Will early treatment cause arrested immunity?
Educational prevention and control programs	Stimulate public awareness of risk factors and behaviors that lead to infection Public awareness of mode of transmission and general practices to prevent or avoid infection	Low compliance with guidelines Historically has been unsuccessful due to socioeconomic and behavioral issues
Vaccine	Prevents infection and disease, cost effective and can make worldwide impact	Not available. A human vaccine remains an elusive goal in design and efficacy

the proposed or executed control and prevention measures are now known to be either very challenging to develop, impractical to execute or ineffectual to control the endemicity and spread of chlamydial ocular, genital or respiratory infections in the human population [27–29]. Table 1 summarizes these control and prevention measures, their advantages and limitations. It is important to point out that results from the measures executed so far have led to the current medical opinion that the vaccine option will likely represent the most reliable and cost effective means to achieve the greatest impact [21, 30] for a number of reasons: first, the mass screening and treatment, or mass and targeted population treatment with antibiotics such as azithromycin have not produced the desired long-term result to eliminate chlamydial ocular or genital infections [27, 29]; second, although chlamydial infections are treatable with antibacterial agents if detected early (e.g. use of tetracycline derivatives, especially doxycycline, and the macrolides or azalides including erythromycin and azithromycin [21]), the high proportion of asymptomatic infections often lead to severe and sometimes irreversible complications, usually presenting as the first symptoms of an infection [30, 31]. In addition, it has been reported that a significant proportion of treated infections may lead to persistence [32, 33], casting doubt on the long-term value of certain chemotherapies. Moreover, most other prevention strategies have economic, convenience and acceptance issues. Furthermore, computer modeling has predicted that a partially protective chlamydial vaccine that prevents certain severe sequelae in a vaccination program would constitute an acceptable short-term goal [34]. Thus, with epidemiologic data indicating persisting and sometimes increasing incidence of ocular and genital *C. trachomatis* infections in the human population worldwide, the urgency for an efficacious vaccine cannot be over emphasized. Unfortunately there is no acceptable human chlamydial vaccine to date due to a number of challenges, ranging from safety considerations through insufficient immunogenicity of vaccine candidates and lack of effective delivery systems, to how to induce long-term immunity (discussed below).

Chlamydia Vaccine Design Requirements and Challenges

Historical Considerations

From the time of early attempts at diagnosis, associations with ocular, genital and respiratory diseases in humans and animals [35–38], and etiologic proof by reinoculation of normal human hosts in the eye with culture isolated chlamydiae [39], the use of an effective vaccine prophylaxis against chlamydial infection and disease has been an important consideration for prevention. Some of the early questions bordered on whether vaccines could be designed separately for ocular, genital and respiratory infections, or for the entire *Chlamydia* genus, members of a species, or subspecies and serotypes (also called serovars or genovars). The valid case for separate approaches to designing human versus veterinary chlamydial vaccines was settled when animal vaccines that prevented specific chlamydial diseases were easily achieved by conventional vaccination methods [40]. Veterinary *Chlamydia* vaccines consisting of live attenuated or inactivated *C. psittaci* strains have been developed and used successfully to protect ewes from chlamydia-induced abortion [25, 41]. The successful animal *Chlamydia* vaccines in current veterinary use consist of live-attenuated or fixed elementary bodies of *C. psittaci* feline strains, which protect against *Chlamydia*-induced abortion in ewes or feline pneumonic chlamydial disease, respectively [25, 40, 41]. Although the successful veterinary vaccines do not prevent infectivity and lack the rigorous immunization schedules, efficacy, safety and toxicity standards of a human vaccine, their efficacy would suggest that a safe and efficacious human vaccine is a possibility. Also, the veterinary chlamydial vaccine success story provides the impetus and hope for future live attenuated human vaccines if the suspected immunopathogenic concerns are alleviated. Unfortunately, despite the successful animal vaccines, early efforts in human vaccines met with considerable challenges that have persisted to date [42–45]. The challenges facing human chlamydial vaccine design first came to light in the early attempts to use basic vaccinology methods to develop a vaccine against trachoma. Thus, whole organism-based vaccines derived by formalin inactivation of culture- or chick embryo-grown EBs, when delivered intramuscularly in alum or mineral oil adjuvant into children in trachoma-endemic areas of Taiwan, East Africa (Ethiopia), northern India and The Gambia in Africa produced mixed and some alarming results [46–52]. Depending on the trial, the results included a transient or temporary decline in trachoma in some vaccinated groups compared to placebo controls, more severe trachoma in some prevaccinated children compared to controls and serovar-specificity of protection where observed [50]. The apparently disappointing outcome of these early vaccine trials that used the intact bacterium and the possibility that the whole chlamydiae contain components that induce both immunoprotective and immunopathogenic immune responses discouraged further effort toward whole organism-based vaccines. But these early vaccine experiences resulted in an expansion of in vivo and in vitro analyses of chlamydial biology into a set of new objectives that remain valid today. These new objectives included the identification of candidate immunopathogenic components of chlamydiae that may at least partly induce the pathogenesis of the sequelae of chlamydial infection and the design of genetic tools to identify and possibly remove the toxic components from the intact organism [53].

Thus, the early disappointing experience with whole organism-based vaccines, the lack of knowledge of the identity of the immunopathogenic components, and the absence of tools to genetically detoxify or modify the intact bacterium and produce safe attenuated strains have combined to dramatically shift the focus of contemporary chlamydial vaccine research in favor of unraveling the basic immunobiology of chlamydial infection. The central objectives are to define and characterize: (1) the elements of the immune response that mediate protection and the associated antimicrobial mechanisms, (2) the candidate vaccine antigens and (3) the immunization and immunomodulatory requirements for inducing long-term immunity in ocular, genital and respiratory mucosae.

Contemporary Vaccine Approaches
Despite the early disappointing results from chlamydial vaccine trials, there is considerable optimism fueling current efforts in vaccine development. The rational basis for optimism for a realistic chlamydial vaccine include: first, clinical and experimental results suggesting that infected individuals or animal models of experimentally induced ocular or genital infections develop a measurable level of protective immunity. Thus, newly infected individuals are less likely to be reinfected, at least by the same serovar [54], resistance to trachoma increases with age [55] and vaccination with inactivated organisms produces a short-lived protection against ocular rechallenge [47]. Also, experimental vaccination and challenge studies in several animal models of genital, respiratory and ocular chlamydial infections, using diverse immunization regimens, have shown that a certain degree of protection characterized by a reduction in infection or prevention of certain complications such as acute inflammation and infertility could be achieved [56–59]. In addition, there is strong evidence that a partial short-lived chlamydial immunity develops after a natural genital infection [54]. Besides, successful veterinary vaccines have been produced that prevented sequelae such as chlamydia-induced abortion and pneumonic chlamydial disease [25, 40, 41]. These findings have provided the impetus to contemporary *Chlamydia* vaccine efforts to analyze the cellular and molecular bases for protective immunity and define the essential immuno-

logic and antigenic requirements for inducing a protective chlamydial immunity in animal models, which should guide human vaccine design and evaluation.

The shift to contemporary vaccinology methods for chlamydial vaccine design has resulted in research focused on 3 mutually inclusive objectives: (1) to analyze the immunobiology of chlamydial infection in relevant animal models, with supporting clinical studies, to define the immune elements that correlate with protective immunity, and elucidate the antimicrobial mechanisms of the immune effectors; (2) to apply genomics, proteomics, bioinformatics and in vitro and in vivo immunologic techniques to identify stable vaccine candidates, and (3) to utilize modern vaccinology techniques (based on knowledge of factors that regulate immunity at mucosal sites of infection) to boost long-term protective immunity through immunomodulation and development of effective delivery systems and potent adjuvants. Interestingly, considerable progress has been made in the first two objectives but the third objective has remained elusive. As discussed in detail below, the advances in the first two key vaccine objectives (i.e. correlates of protective immunity and vaccine candidates) have culminated in the derivation of specific immunologic paradigms guiding contemporary vaccine design efforts. However, rapid progress is needed on the third objective (i.e. vaccine delivery vehicles) to provide the theoretical basis for designing efficacious vaccines that confer long-lasting immunity against *Chlamydia*.

Correlates of Protective Chlamydial Immunity and Basis of Vaccine Testing
Clinical studies in humans and experimentation in animal infection models have revealed that immunity to *C. trachomatis* correlates with a strong CD4 Th1 response and a complementary antibody response whose function includes fostering a rapid and robust memory T cell-mediated immune (CMI) response during reinfections and possibly the neutralization of infectious particles [56, 58, 60–62]. Thus, as important immunologic correlates for vaccine testing and evaluation, a potentially efficacious vaccine should induce a strong CD4 Th1 response and accessory IgG and IgA antibodies in mucosal and systemic tissues. The antichlamydial action of protective CMI effectors is mediated principally via cytokine-induced antimicrobial mechanisms [56, 58, 60, 63], including a major role for IFN-γ in the cytokine profile of protective cellular effectors, which is reinforced by the genetic evidence for a crucial role of Th1-related cytokines in protective immunity against mycobacterial infections [64]. The biochemical mechanisms of the antimicrobial action of Th1 cytokines include: activation of indoleamine 2,3-dioxygenase (depletion of intracellular tryptophan); activation of inducible nitric oxide synthase (high levels of nitric oxide secretion); deprivation of iron, possibly via downregulation of transferrin receptors, and probably the induction of phagolysosomal fusion or disruption of selective vesicular nutrient transport via p47/GTPase activation [56, 58, 60, 65]. Therefore, chlamydial vaccines inducing these antimicrobial processes are potentially effective. Furthermore, the proposed existence of immunoprotective and immunopathogenic immune responses during chlamydial infection [66] would suggest that immunomodulatory approaches that would favor the

induction of the former and/or prevent the latter are needed for potential vaccines. Unfortunately, vaccine approaches capable of skewing antichlamydial immune responses toward protection and simultaneously prevent immunopathogenic responses are currently unknown; however, recent reports indicated that certain cytokine profiles of antichlamydial immune effectors are critical for preventing immunopathology [67]. In addition, the recent identification of T17-mediated Th1 response as a mostly deleterious immune response [68, 69] could provide a guide among other antigen screening methods for identification of antigens with the potential to induce immunopathology (discussed below).

Potential Chlamydial Vaccine Candidates

The possibility that whole intact chlamydiae harbor pathogenic components [30, 70], and the absence of tools to genetically detoxify or modify them to produce safe attenuated strains make subunit vaccine the current focus of vaccine research. The list of potential subunit vaccines has continued to grow as progress is made in antigen discovery, functional genomics and proteomics, as well as suitable animal models of chlamydial diseases are established. As recently reviewed [45, 71], these vaccine candidates include the 40-, 60- and 15-kDa outer membrane proteins (OMPs) which are encoded by the Omp-1 (omp A), Omp-2 (omp C) and Omp-3 (omp B) genes, respectively [72]. Of these proteins, the 40-kDa Omp-1 antigen (the major OMP, MOMP), has received an enormous amount of attention due to its immunogenicity, immunoaccessibility, abundance (60% of OMP mass), contribution to the structural integrity of the EB, function as a porin, possession of both species- and genus-specific epitopes, and expression during all phases of the developmental cycle [73]. However, the efficacy of MOMP-based vaccines has been limited, due in part to poor immunogenicity, consequently producing only partial protective immunity. Other potential vaccine candidates are the polymorphic OMPs (Pmp) and the conserved PorB family of membrane proteins [72, 74, 75], as well as an ADP/ATP translocase [76], an immunogenic plasmid protein (pgp3) [77], a proteasome/protease-like activity factor (CPAF) [78], a toxin mapped to the plasticity zone of several strains [79], certain members of the chlamydial type III secretory machinery [80], and a number of hypothetical proteins that have been cloned and tested in animal models [81, 82]. A provisional list of patent claims on chlamydial vaccine candidates has also been published [21]. The continuing progress in chlamydial genomics and proteomics, especially with the use of available novel tools for antigen discovery, including immunoproteomic, antigen profiling and generation of active expression libraries [45, 81, 82] will likely expand the pool of vaccine candidates. Comparative structural and immunologic analyses of these antigens should lead to the judicious selection of a single antigen or a combination of immunogens for a multisubunit vaccine. A major advantage of the multiple subunit approach is the potential synergistic immunologic benefit of a combination of epitopes from multiple antigens, which will likely induce a higher frequency of immune effectors that ensures an effective long-lasting immunity. The role of conformation in the vaccine efficacy of candidate protein antigens is yet to be fully established [83]. However, protein folding may determine the availability of crucial T cell epitopes during antigen processing, and the vaccine delivery medium could potentially affect vaccine conformation, immunization and processing. Furthermore, the effect of carbohydrate or lipid modification of vaccine candidates on the immunogenicity and efficacy of a potential chlamydial vaccine is yet to be evaluated in the vaccine efforts. In fact, an idiotypic mimic of chlamydial glycoplipd exoantigen conferred protective immunity in a mouse genital infection model [84], suggesting that a conjugate of glycoplipd exoantigen and possibly MOMP or one of the Pmp proteins may be a promising vaccine.

Moreover, although an efficacious subunit vaccine is the current focus and previous studies have suggested that chlamydial immunity may be serovar specific [50], a chlamydial vaccine candidate with potential to confer genus-specific immunity would be attractive because of the multiple serovar coverage by a single vaccine. Hopefully, such vaccines will be reactive against epitopes on EBs and RBs, so that they are effective against both the EB and RB forms of chlamydiae, which would raise the expectation that they could prevent infectivity as well as disease. Besides, a broad-acting vaccine that targets immune effectors against both the EB and RB forms of chlamydiae would likely prevent the possibility that persisting RBs may act like a Trojan horse that can reactivate and continue the developmental cycle of *Chlamydia* in infected hosts and present as reinfections. The related issues of whether a single, effective human chlamydial vaccine would confer genus versus serovar-specific immunity, be effective against both the EB and RB forms of chlamydiae, and prevent disease (sequelae) or infectivity will probably remain unresolved until contemporary vaccine strategies guide us to identify a suitable protective antigen(s) that is effectively delivered to confer long-lasting immunity against either ocular, genital or respiratory *Chlamydia* disease. Alternatively, modern vaccinology techniques might be used to design an efficacious chlamydial vaccine that accommodates immunodominant epitopes which would ensure immune effectiveness against both RBs and EBs, as well as confer broad crossreactive immunity.

Finally, the proposed existence of immunoprotective and immunopathogenic immune responses during chlamydial infection [66] would suggest that at least some chlamydial antigens may induce both responses or immunopathology only, and therefore need to be 'de-toxified' or removed from any potential vaccine. Among the screening methods for antigen immunotoxicity, the induction of an inappropriate cytokine profile, such as the absence of IFN-γ [67], or the known immunopathogenic IL-17 [68, 69], and possession of potentially pathogenic properties [53, 85–88] are approaches to be considered. In this respect, apart from the lipopolysaccharide with its known endotoxin activity, gene encoded, potentially immunopathogenic antigens described for chlamydiae so far include the heat shock proteins, the DNA primase, chlamydial OmcB proteins, and some newly identified antigens associated with the pathogenesis of reactive arthritis [85–88]. Mechanistically, certain heat shock proteins induce excessive proinflammatory cytokines such as IL-1 with pathologic consequences, whereas chlamydial DNA primase, the 60-kDa cysteine-rich OmcB protein and some hypothetical antigens have been theorized to induce immunopathology by antigenic mimicry [86–88]. The significance of screening for antigen immunotoxicity cannot be over-emphasized, since it is a potential source of yet unknown adverse vaccine effects that have been reported.

Requirements of Delivery Systems for Efficacious Chlamydial Vaccines

The focus of the third chlamydial vaccine research objective has centered on defining the factors that regulate immunity at the mucosal site of infection and development of novel delivery and immunomodulation strategies to boost protective immunity with a subunit vaccine. The current focus on a subunit vaccine and the findings that most experimental vaccines and natural chlamydial infections induced only partial and temporary immunity would suggest that effective delivery systems are needed for chlamydial vaccines. The objective is centered on the principle of vaccinology that poor delivery can prevent the efficacy of the best vaccine candidate. However, the objective to produce effective delivery systems and adjuvants for boosting mucosal immune responses against chlamydial infections has remained elusive. As an operational definition, delivery system is used contextually in this review to indicate both delivery vectors and delivery vehicles. The requirement for effective delivery in vaccine efficacy includes the need to furnish the necessary immunomodulation to boost effectors and targeting them to appropriate effector sites [89], and the need suggested from findings in previous attempts to deliver candidate subunit vaccines in animal models, which can be summarized as in the following paragraphs.

First, the vast majority of the delivery vehicles used to deliver chlamydial antigens so far have produced mixed results in various animal models [56, 63, 89, 90]. Interestingly, only the IL-10-deficient dendritic cell (DC)-based cellular vaccine produced a sterilizing, long-term immunity in a mouse genital infection model; this immunity correlated with the capacity to induce a high frequency of specific Th1 cells and elevated titers of the CMI-associated IgG2a and IgA antibodies [60]. Chlamydia-pulsed IL-10-deficient DCs appear to possess the necessary antigenic, costimulatory and immunomodulatory machinery for inducing an optimal protective immunity. While the protective cellular vaccine approach is probably of limited practical application for a widespread infection such as *Chlamydia*, it furnishes a benchmark for evaluating other potential vaccines, and its further analysis may guide efforts toward designing a more effective delivery vehicle(s). The efficacy of the system indicates that, given optimal conditions, a protective chlamydial vaccine is possible, and given an effective delivery vehicle, inactivated chlamydial elementary bodies possess sufficient immunogenic epitopes to elicit a protective immunity. It has been suggested that the high efficacy of the DC-based cellular vaccine makes them 'natural adjuvants or preeminent delivery vehicles', useful as tools to guide the design of effective delivery systems

Table 2. Requirements of a potentially efficacious *Chlamydia* vaccine

Vaccine parameter	Preference	Role and effect
Vaccine antigen(s)/ candidate(s)	Subunit vaccine or nontoxic intact chlamydiae (inactivated or live-attenuated)	Ensures vaccine is devoid of potential immunopathogenic components
Immunogenicity profile	A robust protective CD4-driven Th1 response and the accessory antibody response	Ensures the elimination of intracellular chlamydiae
Immunomodulation	Use of effective delivery system/vehicles and mucosal adjuvants to boost memory immune responses against *Chlamydia* in ocular, genital and respiratory mucosae.	Ensures an adequate and long-lasting protective immunity in mucosal sites of chlamydial infection

that mimic the action of DCs, for immunizing against chlamydial infections and to unravel the necessary vaccine machinery in terms of antigens, delivery, immunity and homing requirements [59, 60, 91]. The challenge for vaccinology, therefore, is to develop a delivery system that will mimic the superior immunostimulatory properties of IL-10-deficient DCs to achieve an effective chlamydial vaccine. It is noteworthy that rapid maturation of *Chlamydia*-pulsed IL-10-deficient DCs was a major factor in the acquisition of efficient antigen-presenting cell competence [92].

Second, a list of potential delivery systems and adjuvants for chlamydial vaccine and the effectiveness of some of them in promoting the induction of protective chlamydial immunity has been recently reviewed [89]. They include viral and bacterial vectors (e.g. live poliovirus and vaccinia; or nonliving bacterial ghosts), cellular delivery vehicles (e.g. antigen-presenting cells, APCs, such as DCs), immunomodulators (e.g. cytokines and antibodies), detergent-based vehicles (e.g. ISCOMS), microbial-related components (e.g. CpG-rich oligos, ospA, cholera toxin, complete Freund's adjuvant), adjuvant systems and DNA-based expression plasmids [89, 93]. Table 2 summaries the requirements for designing a potentially efficacious *Chlamydia* vaccine, highlighting the key antigenic, immune and delivery-immunomodulatory issues. The continued application of these delivery systems and others such as virus-like particles and vault nanoparticles [89, 90] may lead to the design of a vaccine with acceptable levels of protective immunity in humans in the near future.

New Paradigms and Strategies for Design and Delivery of Effective Chlamydial Vaccines

Progress made in the analysis of the immunobiology of chlamydial infection in animal models and humans and results from testing experimental vaccines and antigens in animals, has crystallized into immunologic, antigenic and immunomodulatory paradigms for designing efficacious chlamydial vaccines [60, 89] that currently guide vaccine design research. According to these operational paradigms, the design of potentially efficacious *Chlamydia* vaccines requires: (i) the induction of both T cell and antibody responses, (ii) choice of a safe immunogen, preferably a subunit(s) vaccine candidate and (iii) effective delivery that includes immunomodulatory strategies to boost immune effectors and foster mucosal immunity. The guiding hypothesis is that the design of efficacious chlamydial vaccines requires the innovative integration of efficient delivery of multiple subunits or epitopes with adequate co-stimulation and a favorable cytokine environment to elicit a robust specific Th1 and the accessory antibody responses. Based on this hypothesis, certain experimental vaccine delivery approaches appear to hold promise for potential use in future chlamydial vaccine design, as recently reviewed [89]. Some key strategic points can be made as follows.

Targeting the Common Mucosal Immune System
Design of efficacious chlamydial vaccines requires delivery approaches that will appropriately target and optimize specific mucosal immunity. In this respect, immunomodulatory approaches relating to choice of appropriate routes of vaccine administration that optimize the relevant mucosal immune response against *Chlamydia* are needed. A promising approach involves exploiting the cooperative interaction between the mucosal immune inductive sites (i.e. draining lymphoid tissues containing the primary APCs, such as DC, where an immune response is initiated) and the mucosal immune effector sites (e.g. site of infection or disease) of the common mucosal immune system to produce an optimal vaccine efficacy. The induction of an optimal mucosal immunity requires targeting antigens to the specialized APCs of the mucosa-associated lymphoid tissues (MALT) in specific mucosal inductive sites [94]. MALT includes the nasal-associated lymphoid tissue (NALT), gut-associated lymphoid tissue and bronchus-associated lymphoid tissue (BALT). Although not well defined, MALT is evident as genital mucosa lymphoid tissue or ocular mucosa lymphoid tissue after a local infection or inflammatory reaction in these tissues. The genital, ocular and respiratory tracts that are sites of chlamydial infection are therefore in the common mucosa immune system (CMIS). The compartmentalization of the inductive and effector sites of CMIS allows certain inductive and effector sites to interact effectively to produce an optimal immune response [94]. The efficacy of chlamydial vaccines can therefore be optimized by development of mucosal-compatible delivery vehicles and selection of a route of administration that targets the inductive sites producing high levels of Th1 response in the relevant ocular, genital or respiratory mucosa, depending on the site of chlamydial infection or disease. For example, intranasal immunization with certain experimental chlamydial vaccines resulted in partial genital immunity [83]. Nasal immunization caused rapid generation of immune effectors detectable within days [94] and was superior to vaginal, gastric, peritoneal or rectal immunization for in-

ducing mucosal anti-HIV or anti-HSV responses [94, 95], emphasizing the strong link between NALT, BALT and the genital mucosa. The cellular and molecular basis for this cooperation involves, among others, adhesion molecules, cytokines and chemokines that direct cell trafficking, and distinct homing pathways. The specific biological processes include the induction and retention of T cells in the genital mucosa via the $\alpha4\beta1$-VCAM and the $\alpha4\beta7$-MAdCAM leukocyte adhesion pathways [89, 96]. In this regard, several experimental chlamydial vaccines have been delivered intranasally with appropriate vectors to target immune effectors to the genital tract and produced varying degrees of protective immunity [45, 71, 97–99]. While the results remain mixed due to several reasons, including the antigen and profile of immune effectors induced, the results are promising and provide direction in vaccine research to the most appropriate regimen to achieve the desired goal of an efficacious human vaccine against *Chlamydia*.

Mucosal Synergy as a Strategy to Boost Antichlamydial Vaccines through the Common Mucosal Immune System
A potentially novel approach to chlamydial vaccine delivery is to exploit the likely synergistic effects of a combination of mucosal immunizations that reinforce one another to boost immunity at a desired mucosal site. This mucosal synergy hypothesis will combine the effect of the CMIS with tactical selection of cooperative mucosal inductive sites during immunization to optimize the mucosal immunity at a target effector site. For example, the mucosal synergy hypothesis would predict that the combination of intranasal and either intrarectal or intravaginal immunizations will boost immunity in the genital tract. The testing of the hypothesis will likely await the availability of more safe vaccine antigens and mucosal-compatible delivery vehicles. It is, however, a testable hypothesis.

Conclusion

Ongoing chlamydial vaccine design efforts are guided by the contemporary paradigms that have been derived from the immunobiology of chlamydial ocular, genital and respiratory infections. The immunologic requirement of a potentially efficacious vaccine is the induction of a strong CD4 T cell-driven Th1 response, as well as an accessory antibody response that is vital for a rapid and robust memory response to reinfections. The vaccine antigen(s) can be a single or a multisubunit approach that furnishes ample T and B cell epitopes to induce adequate protective immune responses without immunopathogenic responses. The vaccine delivery vehicle and method provide safe and effective immunomodulation to boost the protective immunity and target immune effectors to the genital, ocular or respiratory mucosal site of infection. Most importantly, a vaccine that confers broadly specific and long-term protective immunity against both infection and disease is the ultimate desire. However, a vaccine that prevents only the development of the serious complications of chlamydial infection (e.g. blinding trachoma, pelvic inflammatory disease, ectopic pregnancy, infertility and pneumonia), although it does not prevent infectivity and initial symptoms, would be an acceptable short-term goal. Considering the epidemiology of the major chlamydial diseases (trachoma and STD), prevention of at least the oculogenital infections and ensuing diseases with safe, cheap and effective vaccines is critically needed.

Acknowledgments

We thank Dr. Claudiu Bandea for reading through the chapter and making suggestions. The conclusions in this article are those of the authors and do not necessarily represent the official position of the Centers for Disease Control and Prevention.

References

1 Schachter J: Infection and disease epidemiology; in Stephens RS (ed): *Chlamydia:* Intracellular Biology, Pathogenesis, and Immunity. Washington, ASM, 1999, pp 139–169.

2 Bush RM, Everett KD: Molecular evolution of Chlamydiaceae. Int J Syst Evol Microbiol 2001;51:203–220.

3 World Health Organisation: Global prevalence and incidence of selected curable sexually transmitted infections: overview and estimates. Geneva, WHO, 2001.

4 Centers for Disease Control and Prevention: Sexually transmitted disease surveillance, 2005 Supplement: *Chlamydia* prevalence monitoring project – annual report 2005. Atlanta, HHS/CDC, 2006.

5 Johnson RE, Newhall WJ, Papp JR, Black CM, Gift TL, Steece R, Markowitz LE, Devine OJ, Walsh CM, Wang S, Gunter DC, Irwin KL, DeLisle S, Berman SM: Screening tests to detect *Chlamydia trachomatis* and *Neisseria gonorrhoeae* infections – 2002. MMWR Recomm Rep 2002;51:1–40.

6 Paavonen J, Wolner-Hanssen P: *Chlamydia trachomatis:* a major threat to reproduction. J Hum Reprod 1989;4:111–124.

7 Stamm WE, Guinan ME, Johnson C, Starcher T, Holmes KK, McCormack WM: Effect of treatment regimens for *Neisseria gonorrhoeae* on simultaneous infection with *Chlamydia trachomatis.* N Engl J Med 1984;310:545–549.

8 Rees E: Treatment of pelvic inflammatory disease. Am J Obstet Gynecol 1980;138:1042–1047.

9 Westrom L, Joesoef R, Reynolds G, Hadgu A, Thompson SE: Pelvic inflammatory inflammatory disease and infertility: a cohort study of 1,844 women with laparoscopically verified disease and 657 control women with normal laparoscopy results. Sex Transm Dis 1992;19:185–192.

10 Centers of Disease Control and Prevention: Sexually transmitted disease surveillance, 2000. Atlanta, CDC, 2001.

11 Nieuwenhuis RF, Ossewaarde JM, Gotz HM, Dees J, Thio HB, Thomeer MGJ, den Hollander JC, Neumann MH, van der Meijden WI: Resurgence of lymphogranuloma venereum in Western Europe: an outbreak of *Chlamydia trachomatis* serovar L2 proctitis in the Netherlands among men who have sex with men. Clin Infect Dis 2004;39:996–1003.

12 Thior I, Diouf G, Diaw IK, Sarr AD, Hsieh CC, Ndoye I, Mboup S, Chen L, Essex M, Marlink R, Kanki P: Sexually transmitted diseases and risk of HIV infection in men attending a sexually transmitted diseases clinic in Dakar, Senegal. Afr J Reprod Health 1997;1:26–35.

13 Wilkinson D, Rutherford G: Population-based interventions for reducing sexually transmitted infections, including HIV infection. Cochrane Databse Syst Rev 2001:CD001220.

14 Monno R, Maggi P, Carbonara S, Sibilio G, D'Aprile A, Costa D, Pastore G: *Chlamydia trachomatis* and *Mycobaterium tuberculosis* lung infection in an HIV-positive homosexual man. AIDS Patient Care STDs 2001;15:607–610.

15 Kilmarx PH, Mock PA, Levine WC: Effect of *Chlamydia trachomatis* coinfection on HIV shedding in genital tract secretion. Sex Transm Dis 2001;28:347–348.

16 Mcclelland RS, Wang CC, Mandaliya K, Overbaugh J, Reiner MT, Panteleeff DD, Lavreys L, Ndinya-Achola J, Bwayo JJ, Kreiss JK: Treatment of cervicitis is associated with decreased cervical shedding of HIV-1. AIDS 2001;15:105–110.

17 Chesson HW, Pinkerton SD: Sexually transmitted diseases and the increased risk for HIV transmission: implications for cost-effectiveness analyses of sexually transmitted disease prevention interventions. J Acquir Immune Defic Syndr 2000;24:48–56.

18 Rotchford K, Strum AW, Wilkinson D: Effect of coinfection with STDs and STD treatment on HIV shedding in genital-tract secretions: systematic review and data synthesis. Sex Transm Dis 2000;27:243–248.

19 Kumar S, Hammerschlag M: Acute respiratory infection due to *Chlamydia pneumoniae*: current status of diagnostic methods. Clin Infect Dis 2007;44: 568–576.

20 Kuo CC, Jackson LA, Campbell LA, Grayston JT: *Chlamydia pneumoniae* (TWAR). Clin Microbiol Rev 1995;8:451–461.

21 Mahdi OS, Byrne GI, Kalayoglu M: Emerging strategies in the diagnosis, prevention and treatment of chlamydial infections. Expert Opin Ther Pat 2001; 11:1253–1265.

22 Gaillat J: Clinical manifestations of *Chlamydia pneumoniae* infections. Revue de Med Interne 1996;17: 987–999.

23 Everett KD: *Chlamydia* and *Chlamydiales*: more than meets the eye. Vet Microbiol 2000;75:109–126.

24 Saikku P, Wang SP, Kleemola M, Brander E, Rusanen E, Grayston JT: An epidemic of mild pneumonia due to an unusual strain of *Chlamydia psittaci*. J Infect Dis 1985;151:832–839.

25 Rodolaki A, Salinas J, Papp J: Recent advances on ovine chlamydial abortion. Vet Res 1998;29:275–288.

26 Nietfeld J: Chlamydial infections in small ruminants. Vet Clin North Am Food Anim Pract 2001;17:301–314.

27 West S: Global elimination of blinding trachoma by 2020: where are we? Ophthalmic Epidemiol 2009;16: 205.

28 Ssemanda E, Munoz B, Harding-Esch E, Edwards T, Mkocha H, Bailey R, Sillah A, Stare D, Mabey D, West S, Team PP: Mass treatment with azithromycin for trachoma control: participation clusters in households. PLoS Negl Trop Dis 2010;4:e838.

29 Brunham R, Rekart M: The arrested immunity hypothesis and the epidemiology of chlamydia control. Sex Transm Dis 2008;35:53–54.

30 Cohen CR, Brunham RC: Pathogenesis of *Chlamydia*-induced pelvic inflammatory disease. Sex Transm Infect 1999;75:21–24.

31 Thein J, Zhao P, Liu H, Xu J, Jha H, Miao Y, Pizzarello L, Tapert L, Schachter J, Mabon M, Osaki-Holm S, Lietman T, Paxton A: Does clinical diagnosis indicate chlamydial infection in areas with a low prevalence of trachoma? Ophthalmic Epidemiol 2002;9: 263–269.

32 Bragina EY, Gomberg MA, Dmitriev GA: Electron microscopic evidence of persistent chlamydial infection following treatment. J Eur Acad Dermatol Venereol 2001;15:405–409.

33 Byrne GI: Chlamydial treatment failures: a persistent problem? J Eur Acad Dermatol Venereol 2001;15: 381.

34 De la Maza MA, De la Maza LM: A new computer model for estimating the impact of vaccination protocols and its application to the study of *Chlamydia trachomatis* genital infections. Vaccine 1995;13:119–127.

35 Budai I: *Chlamydia trachomatis*: milestones in clinical and microbiological diagnostics in the last hundred years: a review. Acta Microbiol Immunol Hung 2007;54:5–22.

36 Sowa J, Collier L: Isolation of trachoma virus from patients in West Africa. J Hyg 1960;58:99–108.

37 Hanna L, Thygeson P, Jawetz E: Elementary body virus isolated from clinical trachoma in California. Science 1959;130:1339–1340.

38 Schachter J: The expanding clinical spectrum of infections with *chlamydia trachomatis*. Sex Transm Dis 1977;4:116–118.

39 Collier L, Duke-Elder S, Jones B: Experimental trachoma produced by cultured virus. Part II. Br J Ophthalmol 1960;44:65–88.

40 Longbottom D, Livingstone M: Vaccination against chlamydial infections of man and animals. Vet J 2006;171:263–275.

41 Chalmers WS, Simpson J, Lee SJ, Baxendale W: Use of a live chlamydial vaccine to prevent ovine enzootic abortion. Vet Rec 1997;141:63–67.

42 Schachter J: Overview of *Chlamydia trachomatis* infection and the requirements for a vaccine. Rev Infect Dis 1985;7:713–716.

43 Schachter J, Dawson CR: The epidemiology of trachoma predicts more blindness in the future. Scand J Infect Dis Suppl 1990;69:55–62.

44 Brunham R, Rey-Ladino J: Immunology of *Chlamydia* infection: implications for a *Chlamydia trachomatis* vaccine. Nat Rev Immunol 2005;5:149–161.

45 Rockey D, Wang J, Lei L, Zhong G: Chlamydia vaccine candidates and tools for chlamydial antigen discovery. Expert Rev Vaccines 2008;8:1365–1377.

46 Grayston JT, Woolridge RL, Wang S, Yen C, Yang C, Cheng K, Chang I: Field studies of protection from infection by experimental trachoma virus vaccine in preschool-aged children on Taiwan. Proc Soc Exp Biol Med 1963;112:589–595.

47 Woolridge RL, Grayston JT, Chang IH, Yang CY, Cheng KH: Long-term follow-up of the initial (1959–1960) trachoma vaccine field trial on Taiwan. Am J Ophthalmol 1967;63:1650–1655.

48 Wang SP, Grayston JT, Alexander ER: Trachoma vaccine studies in monkeys. Am J Ophthalmol 1967; 63:1615–1620.

49 Clements C, Dhir S, Grayston J, Wang S: Long term follow-up study of a trachoma vaccine trial in villages of northern India. Am J Ophthalmol 1979;87: 350–353.

50 Grayston JT, Wang SP, Yang YF, Woolridge RL: The effect of trachoma virus vaccine on the course of experimental trachoma infection in blind human volunteers. J Exp Med 1962;115:1009–1022.

51 Bietti G, Guerra P, Vozza R, et al: Results of large-scale vaccination against trachoma in East Africa (Ethiopia) 1960–1965. Am J Ophthalmol 1966;61: 1010–1029.

52 Sowa S, Sowa J, Collier L, Blyth W: Trachoma vaccine field trials in The Gambia. J Hyg (Lond) 1969; 67:699–717.

53 Byrne G: *Chlamydia trachomatis* strains and virulence: rethinking links to infection prevalence and disease severity. J Infect Dis 2010;201:S126–S133.

54 Katz BP, Batteiger BE, Jones RB: Effect of prior sexually transmitted disease on the isolation of *Chlamydia trachomatis*. Sex Transm Dis 1987;14:160–164.

55 Bailey R, Duong T, Carpenter R, Whittle H, Mabey D: The duration of human ocular *Chlamydia trachomatis* infection is age dependent. Epidemiol Infect 1999;123:479–486.

56 Morrison RP, Caldwell HD: Immunity to murine chlamydial genital infection. Infect Immun 2002;70: 2741–2751.

57 de la Maza LM, Peterson EM: Vaccines for *Chlamydia trachomatis* infections. Curr Opin Investig Drugs 2002;3:980–986.

58 Loomis PW, Starnbach MN: T cell responses to *Chlamydia trachomatis*. Curr Opin Microbiol 2002; 5:87–91.

59 Igietseme JU, Black CM, Caldwell HD: Chlamydia vaccine: strategies and status. BioDrugs 2002;16:19–35.

60 Igietseme JU, Eko FO, Black CM: Contemporary approaches to designing and evaluating vaccines against *Chlamydia*. Expert Rev Vaccines 2003;2:129–146.

61 Igietseme JU, Eko FO, He Q, Black CM: Antibody regulation of T cell immunity: implications for vaccine strategies against intracellular pathogens. Expert Rev Vaccines 2004;3:23–34.

62 Cohen CR, Koochesfahani KM, Meier AS, Shen C, Karunakaran K, Ondondo B, Kinyari T, Mugo NR, Nguti R, Brunham RC: Immunoepidemiologic profile of *Chlamydia trachomatis* infection: importance of heat-shock protein 60 and interferon-γ. J Infect Dis 2005;192:591–599.

63 Rank RG: Models of immunity; in Stephens RS (ed): *Chlamydia*: intracellular biology, pathogenesis and immunity. Washington, ASM Press, 1999, pp 239–295.

64 Fieschi C, Casanova J: The role of interleukin-12 in human infectious diseases: only a faint signature. Eur J Immunol 2003;33:1461–1464.

65 Nelson DE, Virok DP, Heidi W, Roshick C, Johnson RM, Whitmire WM, Crane DD, Steele-Mortimer O, Kari L, McClarty G, Caldwell HD: Chlamydia IFN-γ immune evasion is linked to host infection tropism. Proc Natl Acad Sci USA 2005;102:10658–10663.

66 Stephens R: The cellular paradigm of chlamydial pathogenesis. Trends Microbiol 2003;11:44–51.

67 Gondek D, Roan N, Starnbach M: T cell responses in the absence of IFN-γ exacerbate uterine infection with *Chlamydia trachomatis*. J Immunol 2009;183: 1313–1319.

68 Ley K, Smith E, Stark MA: IL-17A-producing neutrophil-regulatory Tn lymphocytes. Immunol Res 2006;34:229–242.

69 Matsuzaki G, Umemura M: Interleukin-17 as an effector molecule of innate and acquired immunity against infections. Microbiol Immunol 2007;51: 1139–1147.

70 LaVerda D, Kalayoglu MV, Byrne GI: Chlamydial heat shock proteins and disease pathology: new paradigms for old problems? Infect Dis Obstet Gynecol 1999;7:64–71.

71 Hafner L, McNeilly C: Vaccines for *Chlamydia* infections of the female genital tract. Future Microbiol 2008;3:67–77.

72 Stephens RS: Chlamydial genomics and vaccine antigen discovery. J Infect Dis 2000;181:S521–S523.

73 Brunham RC, Peeling RW: *Chlamydia trachomatis* antigens: role in immunity and pathogenesis. Infect Agents Dis 1994;3:218–233.

74 Stephens RS, Lammel CJ: Chlamydia outer membrane protein discovery using genomics. Curr Opin Microbiol 2001;4:16–20.

75 Kawa DE, Stephens RS: Antigenic topology of chlamydial PorB protein and identification of targets for immune neutralization of infectivity. J Immunol 2002;168:5184–5191.

76 Murdin AD, Dunn P, Sodoyer R, Wang J, Caterini J, Brunham RC, Aujame L, Oomen R: Use of a mouse lung challenge model to identify antigens protective against *Chlamydia pneumoniae* lung infection. J Infect Dis 2000;181:S544–S551.

77 Donati M, Sambri V, Comanducci M, Di Leo K, Storni E, Giacani L, Ratti G, Cevenini R: DNA immunzation with pgp3 gene of *Chlamydia trachomatis* inhibits the spread of chlamydial infection from the lower to the upper genital tract in C3H/HeN mice. Vaccine 2003;21:1089–1093.

78 Sharma J, Bosnic AM, Piper JM, Zhong G: Human antibody responses to a Chlamydia-secreted protease factor. Infect Immun 2004;72:7164–7171.

79 Belland RJ, Scidmore MA, Crane DD, Hogan DM, Whitmire W, McClarty G, Caldwell HD: *Chlamydia trachomatis* cytotoxicity associated with complete and partial cytotoxin genes. Proc Natl Acad Sci USA 2001;98:13984–13989.

80 Slepenkin A, de la Maza LM, Peterson EM: Interaction between components of the type III secretion system of Chlamydiaceae. J Bacteriol 2005;187:473–479.

81 Meoni E, Faenzi E, Frigimelica E, Zedda L, Skibinski D, Giovinazzi S, Bonci A, Petracca R, Bartolini E, Galli G, Agnusdei M, Nardelli F, Buricchi F, Norais N, Ferlenghi I, Donati M, Cevenini R, Finco O, Grandi G, Grifantini R: CT043, a protective antigen that induces a CD4+ Th1 response during *Chlamydia trachomatis* infection in mice and humans. Infect Immun 2009;77:4168–4176.

82 Follmann F, Olsen A, Jensen K, Hansen P, Andersen P, Theisen M: Antigenic profiling of a *Chlamydia trachomatis* gene-expression library. J Infect Dis 2008;197:897–905.

83 Pal S, Theodor I, Peterson EM, de la Maza LM: Immunization with the *Chlamydia trachomatis* mouse pneumonitis major outer membrane protein can elicit a protective immune response against a genital challenge. Infect Immun 2001;69:6240–6247.

84 Whittum-Hudson JA, Rudy D, Gerard H, Vora G, Davis E, Haller PK, Prattis SM, Hudson AP, Saltzman WM, Stuart ES: The anti-idiotypic antibody to chlamydial glycolipid exoantigen (GLXA) protects mice against genital infection with a human biovar of *Chlamydia trachomatis*. Vaccine 2001;19:4061–4071.

85 Bachmaier K, Neu N, de la Maza LM, Pal S, Hessel A, Penninger JM: *Chlamydia* infections and heart disease linked through antigenic mimicry. Science 1999;283:1335–1339.

86 Bachmaier K, Penninger J: Chlamydia and antigenic mimicry. Curr Top Microbiol Immunol 2005;296: 153–163.

87 Swanborg R, Boros D, Whittum-Hudson J, Hudson A: Molecular mimicry and horror autotoxicus: do chlamydial infections elicit autoimmunity? Expert Rev Mol Med 2006;8:1–23.

88 Cragnolini J, García-Medel N, de Castro J: Endogenous processing and presentation of T cell epitopes from *Chlamydia trachomatis* with relevance in HLA-B27-associated reactive arthritis. Mol Cell Proteomics 2009;8:1850–1859.

89 Igietseme JU, Eko FO, He Q, Bandea C, Lubitz W, Garcia-Sastre A, Black C: Delivery of *Chlamydia* vaccines. Expert Opin Drug Deliv 2005;2:549–562.

90 Champion C, Kickhoefer V, Liu G, Moniz R, Freed A, Bergmann L, Vaccari D, Raval-Fernandes S, Chan A, Rome L, Kelly K: A vault nanoparticle vaccine induces protective mucosal immunity. PLoS One 2009; 4:e5409.

91 Citterio S, Rescigno M, Foti M, Granucci F, Aggujaro D, Gasperi C, Matyszak MK, Girolomoni G, Ricciardi-Castagnoli P: Dendritic cells as natural adjuvants. Methods 1999;19:142–147.

92 He Q, Moore TT, Eko FO, Lyn D, Ananaba GA, Martin A, Singh S, Lillard J, Stiles J, Black CM, Igietseme JU: Molecular basis for the potency of IL-10-deficient dendritic cells as a highly efficient APC system for activating Th1 response. J Immunol 2005;174: 4860–4869.

93 Igietseme JU, Eko FO, Back CM: *Chlamydia* vaccines: recent developments and the role of adjuvants in future formulations. Expert Rev Vaccines 2010;10: 1585–1596.

94 Wu HY, Russell MW: Nasal lymphoid tissue, intranasal immunization, and compartmentalization of the common mucosal immune system. Immunol Res 1997;16:187–201.

95 Staats HF, Montgomery SP, Palker TJ: Intranasal immunization is superior to vaginal, gastric, or rectal immunization for induction of systemic and mucosal anti-HIV antibody responses. AIDS Res Hum Retroviruses 1997;13:945–952.

96 Kelly KA, Rank RG: Identification of homing receptors that mediate the recruitment of CD4 T cells to the genital tract following intravaginal infection with *Chlamydia trachomatis*. Infect Immun 1997;65: 5198–5208.

97 He Q, Martinez-Sobrido L, Eko FO, Palese P, Garcia-Sastre A, Lyn D, Okenu D, Bandea C, Ananaba GA, Black CM, Igietseme JU: Live-attenuated influenza viruses as delivery vectors for *Chlamydia* vaccines. Immunology 2007;122:28–37.

98 Li W, Murthy A, Guentzel M, Seshu J, Forsthuber T, Zhong G, Arulanandam B: Antigen-specific CD4+ T cells produce sufficient IFN-γ to mediate robust protective immunity against genital *Chlamydia muridarum* infection. J Immunol 2008;180:3375–3382.

99 Pal S, Theodor I, Peterson EM, de l Maza LM: Immunization with an acellular vaccine consisting of the outer membrane complex of *Chlamydia trachomatis* induces protection against a genital challenge. Infect Immun 1997;65:3361–3369.

Dr. Joseph U. Igietseme, PhD
National Center for Emerging Zoonotic and Infectious Diseases
Centers for Disease Control and Prevention
1600 Clifton Road NE, Mailstop G36, Atlanta, GA 30333 (USA)
E-Mail Jigietseme@cdc.gov

Black CM (ed): Chlamydial Infection: A Clinical and Public Health Perspective.
Issues Infect Dis. Basel, Karger, 2013, vol 7, pp 131–141 (DOI: 10.1159/000348764)

Maternal and Infant *Chlamydia trachomatis* Infections

Ingrid G.I.J.G. Rours[a] · Margaret R. Hammerschlag[b]

[a]Department of Pediatrics, Sophia Children's Hospital, Erasmus MC University Medical Center, Rotterdam,
The Netherlands; [b]Division of Pediatric Infectious Diseases, Departments of Pediatrics and Medicine, SUNY
Downstate Medical Center, Brooklyn, N.Y., USA

Abstract

Chlamydia trachomatis infections in pregnancy present several challenges. In addition to potentially affecting the pregnancy, the infection may also affect the developing fetus and be transmitted to the infant during parturition. *C. trachomatis* infection during pregnancy has been associated with a number of adverse outcomes including stillbirth, low birth weight and premature delivery. Data on the effect of treatment of maternal infection on outcome of pregnancy have been inconclusive. *C. trachomatis* infection has also been associated with postpartum endometritis and postabortal pelvic inflammatory disease. The risk of an infant born to an infected mother of acquiring *C. trachomatis* infection is approximately 50%. The infant may become infected at multiple sites including the conjunctivae, nasopharynx, rectum and vagina. The most common clinical manifestation is neonatal conjunctivitis. Although the nasopharynx is the most frequent site of infection in infants, most of these infections are asymptomatic and may persist for months. Approximately 25% of infants with nasopharyngeal infection may develop a characteristic pneumonia, usually 1–3 months after birth. The most effective approach to preventing perinatal chlamydial infection is screening and treatment of pregnant women. This has been greatly facilitated by the use of nucleic acid amplification tests for diagnosis and the availability of effective single-dose antibiotic treatment.

The Effect of Pregnancy on *Chlamydia trachomatis* Infection

Various changes in pregnancy have been proposed to influence *C. trachomatis* infection [1]. Cervical ectopy (related to estrogen levels), associated with *C. trachomatis* infection and pregnancy, may increase shedding of *C. trachomatis* and/or increase the risk of chlamydial infection [2]. Furthermore, pregnancy is physiologically immunosuppressive and alters the immune responses progressively with advancing gestation, which may affect replication and shedding of *C. trachomatis*.

The Effect of *C. trachomatis* Infection on Pregnancy

In the First Trimester
C. trachomatis has been associated with spontaneous (recurrent) abortions, though not consistently [3–8]. Various models have been proposed for the pathogenesis of chlamydia-related spontaneous abortions, being either direct zygote infection or an immune response to heat shock proteins expressed by the zygote that is triggered by previous *C. trachomatis* infection, and reactivation of latent chlamydial infection or endometrial damage from past chlamydial infection [3, 6].

In the Second and Third Trimester
Premature Rupture of Membranes, Premature Delivery, Prematurity
C. trachomatis infection during pregnancy may influence pregnancy outcome and has been associated with chorioamnionitis, premature rupture of the membranes and premature delivery [9–24]. However, the literature regarding these effects of *C. trachomatis* infection on pregnancy outcome is conflicting, which seems to be primarily due to differences in the study design, population and microbiological tests that were used. While earlier studies based on serology and cultures were at variance regarding premature delivery, studies that used nucleic acid amplification tests (NAATs) for diagnosis were more likely to find an association of prematurity with *C. trachomatis* infection [19–21].

Low Birth Weight
C. trachomatis infection during pregnancy has been associated with low birth weight. However, again the literature is contradictory and other studies could not confirm such an association, probably also due to heterogeneity of the methods used [21, 25]. In some studies an association of *C. trachomatis* infection with low birth weight could only be confirmed in subgroups of women with elevated anti-*C. trachomatis* IgM antibodies, which suggested acute infection [11, 26]. A major confounding variable in many of these studies was coinfection with other organisms also associated with chorioamnionitis and low birth weight, including genital mycoplasmas, *Trichomonas vaginalis* and bacteria responsible for bacterial vaginosis [25]. The Vaginitis in Pregnancy study, which was a large US multicenter study sponsored by the National Institutes of Health in the early 1990s generated much of these data [24, 25]. A total of 13,750 women were enrolled and *C. trachomatis* was isolated by culture from 1,239 (9%). The Vaginitis in Pregnancy study also included a placebo-controlled study of erythromycin for treatment of *C. trachomatis* infection in pregnant women to determine whether treatment would lower the incidence of preterm delivery and/or low birth weight. The results were equivocal, erythromycin treatment had little impact on reducing low birth weight (defined as <2,500 g) or preterm delivery. There was a 20% failure rate in the erythromycin group which was associated with a higher rate of low birth weight and preterm delivery. However, 37% of women in the placebo group

cleared the infection spontaneously; women in the placebo group were also more likely to use nontrial antibiotics that also had activity against *C. trachomatis* (clindamycin, amoxicillin), which further complicated the analysis.

Stillbirth

C. trachomatis has been implicated as a cause of in utero infection in the fetus leading to stillbirth [10] and again results of various studies have been contradictory. IgM antibodies to *C. trachomatis* can be detected in cord blood of prematurely born neonates, which was felt to be suggestive of fetal infection. However, cord blood can often be contaminated with maternal blood, thus the antibody may be of maternal origin.

Postpartum Effects of *C. trachomatis* Infections

C. trachomatis infection during pregnancy may continue after delivery and cause postpartum endometritis, salpingitis or pelvic inflammatory disease [27–30]. In contrast to early postpartum endometritis, *C. trachomatis* usually causes late postpartum endometritis and develops between 2 days and 6 weeks after delivery [27–30]. Women are usually not seriously ill, but may present with secondary postpartum hemorrhage, with or without fever, lower abdominal pain and vaginal discharge. *C. trachomatis* infection can spread into the fallopian tubes resulting in salpingitis and increasing the risk of infertility or ectopic pregnancy.

C. trachomatis Infections in Newborn Infants

At the time of delivery, newborns may acquire *C. trachomatis* infection from pregnant women during passage through an infected birth canal. Hence, the occurrence of *C. trachomatis* infection in infants is directly related to the prevalence of maternal infection [31–34]. Infants born by caesarean section are at lower risk of acquiring chlamydial infection; however, several anecdotal reports of *C. trachomatis* infections in newborns after delivery by caesarean section, with and without premature rupture of the membranes, indicate that intrauterine infection can occur [35–37]. The overall risk for infants born to women with untreated chlamydial infections is approximately 50–75%, with infection occurring at one or more anatomic sites, including the conjunctivae, nasopharynx, rectum and vagina (table 1). Most of these studies were conducted in the 1980s before maternal screening was mandated in the USA and other developed countries. Approximately 30–50% of infants born to mothers with active, untreated chlamydial infection develop clinical conjunctivitis [31–34, 38]. The nasopharynx is the most frequent site of infection with 78% of infected infants having positive nasopharyngeal cultures in one study [38]. At least 50% of infants with chlamydial conjunctivitis also have nasopharyngeal infection. A recent study from China

Table 1. Selected studies of perinatal chlamydial infection

Study	Prevalence of maternal		proportion of infants with chlamydial infection born to infected mothers				
	chlamydial infection						
	total n	infected n	total n	conjunc-tivitis	pneumonia	NP	rectum/vagina
Frommell et al. [33], 1979, Denver	340	30 (8.8%)	17	39%	11%	6%	NS
Schachter et al. [32], 1986, San Francisco	5,531	262 (4.7%)	131	17.6%	16%	11.5%	14%
Hammerschlag et al. [34], 1989, Brooklyn	4,357	341 (7.8%)	45	15%	1%	4%	NS
Yu et al. [19], 2010, Chongquin, China	300	33 (11%)	8	NS	NS	24.2%	NS

NP = Nasopharnyx; NS = not studied.

documented nasopharyngeal infection, using PCR, in 24.2% of infants born to chlamydia-positive mothers [19]. However no details were given on when the infants were tested or if they were followed or treated. The overall risk of developing pneumonia among infants born to chlamydia-positive mothers has been reported to range from 1 to 22% but only about 25% of infants with nasopharyngeal chlamydial infection develop pneumonia [31–34, 38]. Data on the risk of acquiring rectal or vaginal infection are more limited. Bell et al. [39] demonstrated that perinatally acquired *C. trachomatis* infection may persist for months to years. Twenty-two infants born to women with culture-documented chlamydial infection were followed and positive cultures from the nasopharynx and oropharynx in the infants were detected as late as 28.5 months after birth. Rectal and vaginal infections were asymptomatic and persisted for at least 1 year. This can become an important confounding variable when young children are tested for the presence of *C. trachomatis* during evaluation for suspected sexual abuse.

Before the introduction of systematic prenatal screening for *C. trachomatis* infection and treatment of pregnant women, *C. trachomatis* was probably the most frequent infectious cause of neonatal conjunctivitis in the USA [32]. Since screening and treatment were initiated the incidence of both neonatal conjunctivitis and pneumonia have decreased dramatically. However, in countries where prenatal screening is not done, *C. trachomatis* remains an important cause of neonatal infection, including conjunctivitis. A retrospective/prospective study from the Netherlands demonstrated that *C. trachomatis* was responsible for 61% of cases of neonatal conjunctivitis in infants presenting to a pediatric hospital and ophthalmologists in Rotterdam [40]. Prevalence of *C. trachomatis* infection among pregnant women in that population was 4%; however, prenatal screening and treatment is not standard practice in the Netherlands. Similar data were reported from Ireland, between July 2002 and December 2006, 17 cases of neonatal conjunctivitis due to *C. trachomatis* and one due to *Neisseria gonorrhoeae* were identified in infants presenting to a major Irish regional teaching hospital [41]. The incidence of chlamydial ophthalmia was 0.65/1,000 live births and was found to be rising annually, reflecting the overall increase in genital chlamydial infection in the region. Prenatal screening and treatment for *C. trachomatis* and *N. gonorrhoeae* is not standard practice in Ireland. Yip et al. [42] reported an incidence of neonatal chlamydial conjunctivitis of 4/1,000 live births in Hong Kong over a 12-month period from 2004 to 2005; prenatal screening and treatment are also not standard practice in Hong Kong.

C. trachomatis pneumonia develops in only about 25% of infants with nasopharyngeal infection. In those infants who develop pneumonia, the presentation and clinical findings are very characteristic [43, 44]. The children usually present between 4 and 12 weeks of age. A few cases have been reported presenting as early as 2 weeks of age, but no cases have been seen beyond 4 months. The infants frequently have a history of cough and congestion with an absence of fever. On physical examination the infant is tachypneic, and rales are heard on auscultation of the chest; wheezing is distinctly uncommon [43, 44]. There are no specific radiographic findings except hyperinflation. Significant laboratory findings include peripheral eosinophilia (>300 cells/cm^3) and elevated serum immunoglobulins. If cultured, infants with *C. trachomatis* pneumonia may remain symptomatic and shed the organism from the nasopharynx for protracted periods [38, 43, 44]. Generally, infantile pneumonia due to *C. trachomatis* appears to be self-limited. Most infants can be managed as outpatients although there are a few reports of severe disease requiring hospitalization and assisted ventilation. *C. trachomatis* pneumonia in infants also appears to be associated with few sequelae, although data are limited. Rarely, infants with *C. trachomatis* pneumonia may have concomitant otitis media [43].

Prevention and Control Strategies

Screening of and Treatment of Pregnant Women
Up to 80% of women, including pregnant women, are asymptomatic, hence, they will not seek medical care or perceive themselves as being at risk and may easily be missed while already affected by chlamydial infection or its complications. *C. trachomatis* infection in pregnant women may therefore be an important problem for women and infants, but the extent of the health problem can vary between different populations. By screening during pregnancy, infected women can be identified and treated to reduce the risk of chlamydial disease and its complications for themselves, their offspring and their partners. In the USA, the Centers for Disease Control and Prevention (CDC) has been recommending screening pregnant women for *C. trachomatis* infection at 36 weeks since 1989 [45]. An advantage of screening during pregnancy is that most pregnant women, at least in the developed world and in increasing numbers also in the developing world, spontaneously seek antenatal care. Such visits offer a good opportunity to include a *C. trachomatis* test as part of a routine antenatal care program [46, 47].

Screening should be done with NAATs. Although screening in pregnancy has been recommended in Germany since 1995, the government specified until 2008 that a rapid point-of-care test be used, which resulted in a very low rate of detection – 0.5% in one urban area [48]. These tests have been demonstrated to be very insensitive compared to currently available NAATs [49].

In most countries there is agreement that both symptomatic and asymptomatic pregnant women with *C. trachomatis* infection should be treated considering the possibility of complications. However, therapeutic options are restricted due to the fetus. The teratogenic and embryopathic effects of tetracyclines on bone growth and dentition, interference of doxycycline with normal skeletal growth and increased risk neural tube, cardiovascular and urinary tract defects associated with use of sulfonamides have been described in human and animal studies [50, 51]. The current alternatives for treatment of chlamydial infection in pregnant women include multiple dose treatment with erythromycin, amoxicillin or single-dose treatment with azithromycin [52]. Azithromycin has been shown to be similar or better in treatment success compared to erythromycin and amoxicillin, and to cause similar or less total adverse events and gastrointestinal side effects (nausea, diarrhea, abdominal pain), which resolve spontaneously [53–58]. Azithromycin is currently the first line recommendation by the CDC for the treatment of chlamydial infection during pregnancy [59].

Erythromycin has been shown to be similar or less efficacious than azithromycin, but the long treatment period, multiple dosing regimen and gastrointestinal side effects decrease compliance significantly [52]. In addition, the use of erythromycin in pregnant women and infants has been associated with increased risk for maternal hepatotoxicity and infantile pyloric stenosis [60–63]. Amoxicillin has similar or less efficacy, similar or more reported side effects, and similar or less compliance than azithromycin. In addition, amoxicillin also requires a 7-day treatment period and multiple dosing, but is still a recommended alternative during pregnancy and first choice in some countries, including the Netherlands.

Screening and treatment provides the best option for prevention of infection in the infant. Most of the maternal treatment studies did not follow or evaluate infants for subsequent chlamydial infection. In 1985, McMillan et al. [64] demonstrated in a small study that infants born to women with *C. trachomatis* infection who were treated in the third trimester with erythromycin did not develop either conjunctival or nasopharyngeal infection compared to 23.8% of infants born to infected mothers who received placebo.

Neonatal Ocular Prophylaxis
Neonatal ocular prophylaxis with silver nitrate, topical erythromycin or tetracycline ointment, while effective for prevention of gonococcal ophthalmia, especially in the absence of prenatal screening and treatment, does not prevent chlamydial ophthalmia or nasopharyngeal colonization with *C. trachomatis* or chlamydial pneumonia

[34]. Currently, erythromycin ophthalmic ointment is the only preparation available for neonatal ocular prophylaxis in the USA. Tetracycline ophthalmic ointment is no longer manufactured and silver nitrate has not been available in the USA for almost a decade. New data on efficacy of neonatal ocular prophylaxis and use of other preparations, specifically povidone iodine, are very limited. Four studies of neonatal ocular prophylaxis have been published since 2004, two from Iran, one each from Brazil and Mexico [65–68]. Ali et al. [65] compared Betadine, erythromycin and no prophylaxis in 330 infants in Tehran. Mothers were not tested for *N. gonorrhoeae* or *C. trachomatis* before delivery. There were no cases of gonococcal ophthalmia in any group; the incidence of *C. trachomatis* conjunctivitis in the Betadine, erythromycin and no prophylaxis groups was 22% (2 cases), 14% (1 case) and 14% (1 case), respectively (p = 0.88). Diagnosis of *C. trachomatis* was made by PCR; however, no details were given on the PCR method used. Matinzadeh et al. [66], compared erythromycin to saline in 1,002 infants in Tehran. Mothers were not screened for gonorrhea or *C. trachomatis*. There were no cases of gonococcal ophthalmia, but they did not test for *C. trachomatis*. Ramirez-Ortiz et al. [67] compared 2.5% povidone-iodine and topical chloramphenicol in 2,004 infants in a trachoma-endemic area of southern Mexico. Mothers were not screened prenatally. Diagnosis of *C. trachomatis* infection in the infants was made by in-house PCR. The incidence of *C. trachomatis* conjunctivitis in infants followed up to 16 days after delivery was 1.65% (16 cases) in the chloramphenicol group and 3% (30 cases) in the povidone-iodine group. Silva et al. [68] compared 10% silver nitrate drops and saline in 76 infants in Brazil. Again, prenatal screening for *N. gonorrhoeae* and *C. trachomatis* was not done. Infants were tested at birth, 2 h and 1 week, and followed for 3 months. *C. trachomatis* testing was done by direct fluorescent antibody (DFA) test but the reagent was not specified. There were no cases of gonococcal ophthalmia in either group. However, 20% (8/34) of infants who received silver nitrate and 21% who received saline were positive for *C. trachomatis* at birth, and 23.5% (8/34) and 28.1% (12/42) were positive at 1 week of age. It is very difficult to accurately assess the efficacy of any of the preparations used in these studies as prenatal screening was not done, thus we do not know the prevalence of chlamydial or gonococcal infections in pregnant women in their populations. However, the data presented by Ali et al. [65] and Ramirez-Ortiz et al. [67] suggest that iodine preparations may not be effective for prevention of ophthalmia neonatorum due to either *C. trachomatis* or *N. gonorrhoeae*.

Diagnosis of C. trachomatis Infections in Infants
The 'gold standard' for diagnosis of *C. trachomatis* infections in infants and children has been isolation by culture of *C. trachomatis* from the conjunctiva, nasopharynx, vagina or rectum [69]. Several nonculture tests have been approved for diagnosis of chlamydial conjunctivitis in infants, specifically EIAs and DFAs. The only EIA and DFA assays still available in the USA are Pathfinder® Chlamydia DFA and EIA

Microplate (Bio-Rad Laboratories, Hercules, Calif., USA). These tests appear to perform well with conjunctival specimens with sensitivities greater than or equal to 90% and specificities greater than or equal to 95% compared with culture [69]. Unfortunately, the performance with nasopharyngeal specimens has not been as good, with sensitivities ranging from 33 to 90% [69]. The conjunctiva in infants with chlamydial conjunctivitis is a unique site, easily accessed with very high loads of organisms, thus many nonculture tests will work very well there. Data suggest that PCR is equivalent to culture for detection of *C. trachomatis* in the conjunctiva and nasopharynx of infants with conjunctivitis [70–72]. Hammerschlag et al. [70] evaluated PCR (Amplicor, Roche Molecular Diagnostics, Nutley, N.J., USA) for the detection of *C. trachomatis* in ocular and nasopharyngeal specimens from 75 infants with suspected chlamydial conjunctivitis. Amplicor was equivalent to culture for eye specimens with sensitivity and specificity of 92.3 and 100%, respectively. The sensitivity and specificity for nasopharyngeal specimens was 100 and 97.2%. PCR also detected *C. trachomatis* in the urine of 12 out of 12 mothers of culture-positive infants. One can assume that other available NAATs for *C. trachomatis* will work just as well for conjunctival specimens, although none have been specifically approved for use at this site.

Treatment of Chlamydial Conjunctivitis and Pneumonia in Infants
Oral erythromycin suspension (ethylsuccinate or stearate; 50 mg/kg/day for 14 days) is the therapy of choice for the treatment of chlamydial conjunctivitis and pneumonia in infants [45, 59]. It provides better and faster resolution of the conjunctivitis as well as treating any concurrent nasopharyngeal infection, which prevents the development of pneumonia. Additional topical therapy is not needed. The efficacy of this regimen has been reported to range from 80 to 90%, whilst as many as 20% of infants may require another course of therapy [38]. Erythromycin at the same dose for 2 weeks is the treatment of choice for pneumonia and does result in clinical improvement as well as elimination of the organism from the respiratory tract.

Treatment with oral erythromycin has been associated with infantile hypertrophic pyloric stenosis in infants less than 6 weeks of age who were given the drug for prophylaxis after nursery exposure to pertussis [61–63]. Erythromycin is a motilin receptor agonist. Data on use of other macrolides, including azithromycin or clarithromycin, for the treatment of neonatal chlamydia infection are limited. There are no published studies of clarithromycin and only one small study that evaluated azithromycin which found that a short course of azithromycin suspension, 20 mg/kg/day orally, one dose daily for 3 days, was as effective as 2 weeks of erythromycin in eradication of *C. trachomatis* from the conjunctivae and nasopharynx of infants with conjunctivitis [73].

References

1 Cates W Jr, Wasserheit JN: Genital chlamydial infections: epidemiology and reproductive sequelae. Am J Obstet Gynecol 1991;164:1771–1781.

2 Debattista J, Timms P, Allan J: Immunopathogenesis of *Chlamydia trachomatis* infections in women. Fertil Steril 2003;79:1273–1287.

3 Vigil P, Tapia A, Zacharias S, Riquelme R, Salgado AM, Varleta J: First-trimester pregnancy loss and active *Chlamydia trachomatis* infection: correlation and ultrastructural evidence. Andrologia 2002 ;34: 373–378.

4 Rastogi S, Salhan S, Mittal A: Detection of *Chlamydia trachomatis* antigen in spontaneous abortions. Is this organism a primary or secondary indicator of risk? Br J Biomed Sci 2000;57:126–129.

5 Osser S, Persson K: Chlamydial antibodies in women who suffer miscarriage. Br J Obstet Gynaecol 1996; 103:137–141.

6 Witkin SS, Ledger WJ: Antibodies to *Chlamydia trachomatis* in sera of women with recurrent spontaneous abortions. Am J Obstet Gynecol 1992;167:135–139.

7 Quinn PA, Petric M, Barkin M, Butany J, Derzko C, Gysler M, Lie KI, Shewchuck AB, Shuber J, Ryan E: Prevalence of antibody to *Chlamydia trachomatis* in spontaneous abortion and infertility. Am J Obstet Gynecol 1987;156:291–296.

8 Licciardi F, Grifo JA, Rosenwaks Z, Witkin SS: Relation between antibodies to *Chlamydia trachomatis* and spontaneous abortion following in vitro fertilization. J Assist Reprod Genet 1992;9:207–210.

9 Andrews WW, Klebanoff MA, Thom EA, Hauth JC, Carey JC, Meis PJ, Caritis SN, Leveno KJ, Wapner RJ, Varner MW, Iams JD, Moawad A, Miodovnick M, Sibai B, Dombrowski M, Langer O, O'Sullivan M: Midpregnancy genitourinary tract infection with *Chlamydia trachomatis*: association with subsequent preterm delivery in women with bacterial vaginosis and *Trichomonas vaginalis*. Am J Obstet Gynecol 2006;194:493–500.

10 Gibbs RS: The origins of stillbirth: infectious diseases. Semin Perinatol 2002;26:75–78.

11 Harrison HR, Alexander ER, Weinstein L, Lewis M, Nash M, Sim DA: Cervical *Chlamydia trachomatis* and mycoplasmal infections in pregnancy: epidemiology and outcomes. JAMA 1983;250:1721–1727.

12 Cohen I, Veille JC, Calkins BM: Improved pregnancy outcome following successful treatment of chlamydial infection. JAMA 1990;263:3160–3163.

13 Ryan GM Jr, Abdella TN, McNeeley SG, Baselski VS, Drummond DE: *Chlamydia trachomatis* infection in pregnancy and effect of treatment on outcome. Am J Obstet Gynecol 1990;162:34–39.

14 Alger LS, Lovchik JC, Hebel JR, Blackmon LR, Crenshaw MC: The association of *Chlamydia trachomatis, Neisseria gonorrhoeae,* and group B streptococci with preterm rupture of the membranes and pregnancy outcome. Am J Obstet Gynecol 1988;159:397–404.

15 Sweet RL, Landers DV, Walker C, Schachter J: *Chlamydia trachomatis* infection and pregnancy outcome. Am J Obstet Gynecol 1987;156:824–833.

16 Gravett MG, Nelson HP, DeRouen T, Critchlow C, Eschenbach DA, Holmes KK: Independent associations of bacterial vaginosis and *Chlamydia trachomatis* infection with adverse pregnancy outcome. JAMA 1986;256:1899–1903.

17 Martius J, Krohn MA, Hillier SL, Stamm WE, Holmes KK, Eschenbach DA: Relationships of vaginal *Lactobacillus* species, cervical *Chlamydia trachomatis,* and bacterial vaginosis to preterm birth. Obstet Gynecol 1988;71:89–95.

18 Karinen L, Pouta A, Bloigu A, Koskela P, Paldanius M, Leinonen M, Saikku P, Jêrvelin MR, Hartikainen AL: Serum C-reactive protein and *Chlamydia trachomatis* antibodies in preterm delivery. Obstet Gynecol 2005;106:73–80.

19 Yu J, Wu S, Li F, Hu L: Vertical transmission of *Chlamydia trachomatis* in Chongqing, China. Curr Microbiol 2009;58:315–320.

20 Andrews WW, Goldenberg RL, Mercer B, Iams J, Meis P, Moawad A, Das A, Vanstorsten JP, Caritis SN, Thurnau G, Miodovnik M, Roberts J, McNellis D: The Preterm Prediction Study: association of second-trimester genitourinary chlamydia infection with subsequent spontaneous preterm birth. Am J Obstet Gynecol 2000;183:662–668.

21 Blas MM, Canchihuaman FA, Alva IE, Hawes SE: Pregnancy outcomes in women infected with *Chlamydia trachomatis*: a population-based cohort study in Washington State. Sex Transm Infect 2007;83: 314–318.

22 Odendaal HJ, Schoeman J: The association between *Chlamydia trachomatis* genital infection and spontaneous preterm labour. S Afr J Obstet Gynaecol 2006; 12:146–149.

23 Rastogi S, Das B, Salhan S, Mittal A: Effect of treatment for *Chlamydia trachomatis* during pregnancy. Int J Gynaecol Obstet 2003;80:129–137.

24 Martin DH, Eschenbach DA, Cotch MF, Nugent RP, Rao AV, Klebanoff MA, Lou Y, Rettig PJ, Gibbs RS, Pastoreck JG, Regan JA, Kaslow RA: Double-blind placebo-controlled treatment trial of *Chlamydia trachomatis* endocervical infections in pregnant women. Infect Dis Obstet Gynecol 1997;5:10–17.

25 Germain M, Krohn MA, Hillier SL, Eschenbach DA: Genital flora in pregnancy and its association with intrauterine growth retardation. J Clin Microbiol 1994;32:2162–168.

26 Berman SM, Harrison HR, Boyce WT, Haffner WJ, Lewis M, Arthur JB: Low birth weight, prematurity, and postpartum endometritis: association with prenatal cervical *Mycoplasma hominis* and *Chlamydia trachomatis* infections. JAMA 1987;257:1189–1194.

27 Hoyme UB, Kiviat N, Eschenbach DA: Microbiology and treatment of late postpartum endometritis. Obstet Gynecol 1986;68:226–232.

28 Plummer FA, Laga M, Brunham RC, Piot P, Ronald AR, Bhullar V, Mati JY, Ndinya-Achola JO, Cheang M, Nsanze H: Postpartum upper genital tract infections in Nairobi, Kenya: epidemiology, etiology, and risk factors. J Infect Dis 1987;156:92–98.

29 Temmerman M, Laga M, Ndinya-Achola JO, Paraskevas M, Brunham RC, Plummer FA, et al: Microbial aetiology and diagnostic criteria of postpartum endometritis in Nairobi, Kenya. Genitourin Med 1988;64:172–175.

30 Wager GP, Martin DH, Koutsky L, Eschenbach DA, Daling JR, Chiang WT, Alexander ER, Holmes KK: Puerperal infectious morbidity: relationship to route of delivery and to antepartum *Chlamydia trachomatis* infection. Am J Obstet Gynecol 1980;138:1028–1033.

31 Schachter J, Sweet RL, Grossman M, Landers D, Robbie M, Bishop E: Experience with the routine use of erythromycin for chlamydial infections in pregnancy. N Engl J Med 1986;314:276–279.

32 Schachter J, Grossman M, Sweet RL, Holt J, Jordan C, Bishop E: Prospective study of perinatal transmission of *Chlamydia trachomatis*. JAMA 1986;255:3374–3377.

33 Frommell GT, Rothenberg R, Wang SP, McIntosh K: Chlamydial infection of mothers and their infants. J Pediatr 1979;95:28–32.

34 Hammerschlag MR, Cummings CC, Roblin PM, Williams TH, Delke I: Efficacy of neonatal ocular prophylaxis for the prevention of chlamydial and gonococcal conjunctivitis. New Engl J Med 1989;320:769–772.

35 La Scolea LJ Jr, Paroski JS, Burzynski L, Faden HS: *Chlamydia trachomatis* infection in infants delivered by cesarean section. Clin Pediatr (Phila) 1984;23:118–120.

36 Shariat H, Young M, Abedin M: An interesting case presentation: a possible new route for perinatal acquisition of *Chlamydia*. J Perinatol 1992;12:300–302.

37 Bell TA, Stamm WE, Kuo CC, Wang SP, Holmes KK, Grayston JT: Risk of perinatal transmission of *Chlamydia trachomatis* by mode of delivery. J Infect 1994;29:165–169.

38 Hammerschlag MR, Chandler JW, Alexander ER, English M, Koustky L: Longitudinal studies of chlamydial infection in the first year of life. Pediatr Infect Dis 1982;1:395–401.

39 Bell TA, Stamm WE, Wang SP, Kuo CC, Holmes KK, Grayston JT: Chronic *Chlamydia trachomatis* infections in infants. JAMA 1992;267:400–402.

40 Rours GIJG, Hammerschlag MR, De Faber JTHN, de Groot R, Verkooyen RP: *Chlamydia trachomatis* as a cause of neonatal conjunctivitis in Dutch infants. Pediatrics 2008;121:e321–e326.

41 Quirke M, Cullinane A: Recent trends in chlamydial and gonococcal conjunctivitis among neonates and adults in an Irish hospital. Int J Infect Dis 2008;12:371–373.

42 Yip TP, Chan WH, Yip KT, Que TL, Lee MM, Kwong NS, Ho CK: Incidence of neonatal chlamydial conjunctivitis and its association with nasopharyngeal colonization in a Hong Kong hospital assesses by polymerase chain reaction. Hong Kong Med J 2007;13:22–26.

43 Beem MO, Saxon EM: Respiratory-tract colonization and a distinctive pneumonia syndrome in infants infected with *Chlamydia trachomatis*. N Engl J Med 1977;296:306–310.

44 Harrison HR, English MG, Lee CK, Alexander ER: *Chlamydia trachomatis* infant pneumonitis: comparison with matched controls and other infant pneumonitis. N Engl J Med 1978;298:702–708.

45 Centers for Disease Control and Prevention: Sexually transmitted diseases treatment guidelines. MMWR Recomm Rep 2006;55(RR-11):1–94.

46 Bernloehr A, Smith P, Vydelingum V: Antenatal care in the European Union: a survey on guidelines in all 25 member states of the community. Eur J Obstet Gynecol Reprod Biol 2005;122:22–32.

47 US Preventive Services Task Force: Screening for chlamydial infection: US Preventive Services Task Force recommendation statement. Ann Intern Med 2007;147:128–134.

48 Weissenbacher TM, Kupka MS, Kainer F, Friese K, Mylonas I: Screening for *Chlamydia trachomatis* in pregnancy: a restropseoctive analysis in a German urban area. Arch Gynecol Obstet 2011;283:1343–1347.

49 van Dommelen lL, van Tiel FH, Ouburg S, Brouwers EEHG, Terporten PHW, Savelkoul PHM, Morré SA, Bruggeman CA, Hoebe CJPA: Alarmingly poor performance in *Chlamydia trachomatis* point-of-care testing. Sex Transm Infect 2010;86:355–359.

50 Demers P, Fraser D, Goldbloom RB, Haworth JC, LaRochelle J, MacLean R, Murray TK: Effects of tetracyclines on skeletal growth and dentition. A report by the Nutrition Committee of the Canadian Paediatric Society. Can Med Assoc J 1968;99:849–854.

51 Czeizel AE, Rockenbauer M, Sorensen HT, Olsen J: The teratogenic risk of trimethoprim-sulfonamides: a population based case-control study. Reprod Toxicol 2001;15:637–646.

52 Geisler WM: Management of uncomplicated *Chlamydia trachomatis* infections in adolescents and adults: evidence reviewed for the 2006 Centers for Disease Control and Prevention Sexually Transmitted Diseases Treatment Guidelines. Clin Infect Dis 2007;44(suppl 3):S77–S83.

53 Kacmar J, Cheh E, Montagno A, Peipert JF: A randomized trial of azithromycin versus amoxicillin for the treatment of *Chlamydia trachomatis* in pregnancy. Infect Dis Obstet Gynecol 2001;9:197–202.

54 Pitsouni E, Iavazzo C, Athanasiou S, Falagas ME: Single-dose azithromycin versus erythromycin or amoxicillin for *Chlamydia trachomatis* infection during pregnancy: a meta-analysis of randomised controlled trials. Int J Antimicrob Agents 2007;30: 213–221.

55 Rahangdale L, Guerry S, Bauer HM, Packel L, Rhew M, Baxter R, Chow J, Bolan G: An observational cohort study of *Chlamydia trachomatis* treatment in pregnancy. Sex Transm Dis 2006;33:106–110.

56 Adair CD, Gunter M, Stovall TG, McElroy G, Veille JC, Ernest JM: Chlamydia in pregnancy: a randomized trial of azithromycin and erythromycin. Obstet Gynecol 1998;91:165–168.

57 Wehbeh HA, Ruggeirio RM, Shahem S, Lopez G, Ali Y: Single-dose azithromycin for *Chlamydia* in pregnant women. J Reprod Med 1998;43:509–514.

58 Jacobson GF, Autry AM, Kirby RS, Liverman EM, Motley RU: A randomized controlled trial comparing amoxicillin and azithromycin for the treatment of *Chlamydia trachomatis* in pregnancy. Am J Obstet Gynecol 2001;184:1352–1354.

59 Workowski KA, Berman S, Centers for Disease Control and Prevention: Sexually transmitted diseases treatment guidelines, 2010. MMWR Recomm Rep 2010,59(RR-12):1–110.

60 Howe E, Howe E, Benn RA: Hepatotoxicity due to erythromycin ethylsuccinate. Med J Aust 1993;158: 142–144.

61 Honein MA, Paulozzi LJ, Himelright IM, Lee B, Cragan JD, Patterson L, Correa A, Hall S, Erickson JD: Infantile hypertrophic pyloric stenosis after pertussis prophylaxis with erythromycin: a case review and cohort study. Lancet 1999;354:2101–2105.

62 Mahon BE, Rosenman MB, Kleiman MB: Maternal and infant use of erythromycin and other macrolide antibiotics as risk factors for infantile hypertrophic pyloric stenosis. J Pediatr 2001;139:380–384.

63 Cooper WO, Griffin MR, Arbogast P, Hickson GB, Gautam S, Ray WA: Very early exposure to erythromycin and infantile hypertrophic pyloric stenosis. Arch Pediatr Adolesc Med 2002;156:647–650.

64 McMillan JA, Weiner LB, Lamberson HV, Hagen JH, Aubry RH, Abdul-Karim RW, Sunderji SG, Higgens AP: Efficacy of maternal screening and therapy in the prevention of chlamydia infection in the newborn. Infection 1985;13:263–266.

65 Ali Z, Khadije D, Elahe A, Mohammed M, Fateme Z, Narges Z: Prophylaxis of ophthalmia neonatorum comparison of Betadine, erythromycin and no prophylaxis. J Trop Pediatr 2007;53:388–392.

66 Matinzadeh ZK, Beiragadar F, Kavemanesh Z, Abolgasemi H, Amirsalari S: Efficacy of topical ophthalmic prophylaxis in prevention of ophthalmia neonatorum. Trop Doc 2007;37:47–49.

67 Ramirez-Ortiz MA, Rodriguez-Almaraz M, Ochoa-Diazlopez H, Diaz-Prieto P, Rodriguez-Suárez RS: Randomised equivalency trial comparing 2.5% povidone-iodine drops and ophthalmic chloramphenicol for preventing neonatal conjunctivitisin a trachoma endemic area in southern Mexico. Br J Ophthalmol 2007;91:1430–1434.

68 Silva LR, Gurgel RQ, Lima DRR, Cuevas LE: Current usefulness of Credé's method of preventing neonatal ophthalmia. Ann Trop Pediatr 2008;28:45–48.

69 Rodriguez EM, Hammerschlag MR: Diagnostic methods for *Chlamydia trachomatis* disease in infants. J Perinatol 1987;7:232–234.

70 Hammerschlag MR, Roblin PM, Gelling M, Tsumura N, Jules J, Kutlin A: Use of polymerase chain reaction for the detection of *Chlamydia trachomatis* in ocular and nasopharyngeal specimens from infants with conjunctivitis. Pediatr Infect Dis J 1997;16:293–297.

71 Yip PP, Chan WH, Yip KT, Que TL, Kwong NS, Ho CK: The use of polymerase chain reaction assay versus conventional methods in detecting neonatal chlamydial conjunctivitis. J Pediatr Ophthalmol Strabis 2008;45:234–239.

72 Darville T: *Chlamydia trachomatis* infections in neonates and young children. Sem Pediatr Infect Dis 2005;16:235–244.

73 Hammerschlag MR, Gelling M, Roblin PM, Kutlin A, Jule JE: Treatment of neonatal chlamydial conjunctivitis with azithromycin. Pediatr Infect Dis J 1998;17:1049–1050.

Margaret R. Hammerschlag, MD
Division of Infectious Diseases, Departments of Pediatrics
SUNY Downstate Medical Center
450 Clarkson Avenue, Brooklyn, NY 11203-2098 (USA)
E-Mail mhammerschlag@downstate.edu

Black CM (ed): Chlamydial Infection: A Clinical and Public Health Perspective.
Issues Infect Dis. Basel, Karger, 2013, vol 7, pp 142–150 (DOI: 10.1159/000348766)

Chlamydia trachomatis Infection among Sexual Minorities

Devika Singh · Jeanne M. Marrazzo

Harborview Medical Center, Seattle, Wash., USA

Abstract

Same sex behavior is not infrequent among women in the USA and despite widespread prevalence of chlamydial infections, few data are available that describe its prevalence among these sexual minority communities. Recent studies indicate that some women who have sex with women (WSW) are at increased risk for STDs as a result of reported risk behaviors including sex with high-risk men. WSW should undergo routine age-based annual screening for *Chlamydia trachomatis*, as recommended by Centers for Disease Control and Prevention guidelines. Although incident HIV infection and a number of unsafe sex practices declined from the 1980s into the 1990s, men who report sex with men (MSM) continue to be at high risk for genitourinary and rectal chlamydial infection, and a high proportion of rectal infections are reported to occur in asymptomatic men. For MSM, providers are responsible for taking comprehensive sexual histories, conducting thorough physical exams and testing both urethral and rectal sites for chlamydia. Despite public health efforts, historically few STD clinics and gay men's health centers have offered rectal chlamydial screening for asymptomatic MSM. Implementation of nucleic acid amplification testing at rectal sites has been reported to be highly feasible. Providers should also be aware of risks for lymphogranuloma venereum infection and empirically initiate therapy in the appropriate clinical settings.

According to the 2006–2008 National Survey of Family Growth, 13% of women and 5.2% of men aged 15–44 years reported same sex behavior in their lifetime [1]. Women who have sex with women (WSW) represent diverse communities of women who may exclusively have sex with women, or historically (or currently) engage in sexual partnerships with both men and women. Despite the fact that same sex behavior is not infrequent among women in the USA and despite the widespread prevalence of chlamydia, little data at the clinic, community or population levels are available that describe its prevalence among these sexual minority communities. Numerous studies support that more than 90% of women who self-identify as lesbian report a sexual history with men [2]. Moreover, recent studies indicate that some communities of WSW, particularly adolescents and young women, might be at increased risk for STDs and HIV as a result of certain reported risk behaviors [3–5], including sex with high-risk men.

While incident HIV infection and a number of unsafe sexual practices declined from the 1980s into the 1990s, more recent data suggests that a number of sexually transmitted infections (STIs) are on the rise among men who have sex with men (MSM), including *Chlamydia trachomatis* [6, 7]. A number of high-risk sexual behaviors among some subgroups of MSM appear to be associated with higher rates of STI, including decreased safer sex precautions ('prevention fatigue'), illicit drug use, especially methamphetamine use, dynamic patterns within sexual networks (e.g. meeting sex partners online) that promote more anonymous partnerships and an evolving trend of seeking sexual partners of the same serostatus ('serosorting'). This chapter will explore known and potential risk factors for chlamydial infection and transmission among WSW and MSM.

Women Who Have Sex with Women

Same sex sexual behavior is likely underreported to care providers [8]. Moreover, tremendous gaps of knowledge exist in understanding what specific sexual behaviors among WSW place them at risk for STI. Beyond exploring the sex and number of sex partners of their WSW patients, clinicians should elicit history of past and current sex with men, history of preventive health examinations (including Papanicolaou smears and STI screens), detailed sexual practices (oral sex, anal sex, penetrative sex with toys/objects, etc.), use of safer sex methods (dental dams, condoms, etc.) and associated drug use. Sexual practices involving digital-vaginal or digital-anal contact and those including penetrative sex objects represent plausible means for transmission of cervicovaginal secretions.

Prior studies indicate that women who practice same sex behavior, including exclusively same sex behavior, are at risk for STIs, including genital types of human papillomavirus, HIV, genital herpes and trichomoniasis [9–15]. Moreover, bacterial vaginosis occurs commonly among women who report sex with women, and there is a high degree of concordance among monogamous same sex couples, suggesting a potential role for sexual transmission in this group [16]. These observations emphasize the need for healthcare providers and public health advocates to address the sexual and reproductive health care needs of this group of women in a comprehensive and informed manner.

In the first analysis of its kind, researchers found that women aged 15–24 years attending family planning clinics in the US Pacific Northwest during 1997 through 2005 and who reported same sex behavior had higher positivity of *C. trachomatis* than women who reported exclusively heterosexual behavior [17]. Factors associated with chlamydial infection among WSW in this study included use of nucleic acid amplification tests (NAATs) for diagnosis, testing at a non-'routine visit,' report of genitourinary symptoms and report of a sex partner with chlamydial infection. Over the study period, WSW who reported sexual behavioral risks also had the highest chlamydia positivity compared to women reporting sex only with men or women who reported sex with men and women who reported similar risks. Interestingly, a greater proportion of women reporting sex with men and women reported sexual risk behaviors compared with both heterosexual women and those reporting sex only with women; despite this, *C. trachomatis* positivity was not highest in this group. Of note, researchers also noted relatively high chlamydia positivity among American Indian/Alaska Native women who reported sex with women, a finding that is consistent with racial/ethnic disparities previously described from the Region X IPP data [18]. The finding of higher chlamydia positivity among WSW relative to women reporting sex exclusively with men was unexpected. Possible explanations for this observation relate to differences in these two groups' use of reproductive health care services (including chlamydia screening), biological susceptibility to lower genital tract infection, infrequent use of barrier methods to prevent STI transmission with female partners, trends towards higher risk behaviors and differential characteristics of their respective sexual networks.

Overall, findings of higher chlamydia positivity among WSW and women who have sex with men and women in the study noted above are consistent with previously published research documenting that women who report same sex behavior, including those who report sex only with women, often report a history of STI [19, 20]. Previous analyses of clinic-based data from the USA, UK and Australia have reported detection of chlamydial infection among women reporting sex with women. In one study of 708 new patients attending a sexual health clinic for lesbians in London, fewer WSW than those who reported sex only with men underwent endocervical culture for *C. trachomatis*, but infection was diagnosed in 2 women reporting sex exclusively with women [19].

With regard to access to and use of reproductive health services, several investigators have reported that WSW are less likely to undergo routine Papanicolaou smear screening – and generally, preventive gynecologic care, often sought in the context of obtaining birth control – relative to their exclusively heterosexual counterparts [21, 22]. This would logically reduce the number of healthcare encounters at which chlamydia testing would likely be performed. Moreover, most women who report same sex behavior often do not believe that they are at risk of acquiring STI from their female partners [23]. This may lead to less frequent use of some preventive measures (for example, washing sex toys between partners) or infrequent use of barrier methods (including gloves, condoms, dental dams) for STI prevention [24]. Further, healthcare providers do not always obtain a complete sexual history and may thus fail to elicit reports from WSW of higher risk behaviors that would prompt *C. trachomatis* screening and related prevention counseling [25].

Another potential explanation for findings of some STIs, including chlamydia, among WSW relates to selection of sex partners. Some women who report same sex behavior may be more likely to select higher risk sex partners and participate in higher risk behaviors, including unprotected vaginal and anal sex with homosexual or bisexual men [2, 26]. One large cross-sectional survey across healthcare sites in the USA found that women who identified as lesbians reported more male sex partners and higher numbers of male sex partners who reported sex with other men in the past year than either heterosexual or bisexual women [5]. In a Seattle-based study of women reporting sex with at least 1 woman in the past year, concurrency (overlap between partnerships reported by participant) was common, especially among bisexual women [27]. Moreover, bisexual women frequently reported inconsistent condom use with either vaginal or anal intercourse with men. Many of these women (16%) believed their male partner had sex with another man at some point in time. Additional studies have demonstrated other high-risk behaviors among some WSW, including use of injection drugs and crack cocaine, and exchange of sex for drugs or money [2, 28–31].

Finally, bacterial vaginosis, a condition that occurs when the hydrogen peroxide-producing *Lactobacillus* species that characterizes the normal human vagina are replaced by high quantities of commensal anaerobic bacteria, increases the risk of STI acquisition, including *C. trachomatis* [32–34]. For reasons that are unclear, bacterial vaginosis is highly prevalent in WSW [16, 35–39], and could theoretically place same sex reporting women at increased risk for this infection if sexual exposure to *C. trachomatis* occurs.

Taken together, the data cited above emphasize that WSW should undergo routine age-based annual screening for *C. trachomatis* as recommended by current guidelines, which include annual screening for women younger than 25 years and others at increased risk per the US Preventive Services Task Force [40] or including age 25 years and younger and others at increased risk per the Centers for Disease Control and Prevention (CDC) [41].

Men Who Have Sex with Men

Standard guidelines from the US CDC urge clinicians to sensitively explore STI risk behaviors and review patient-centered prevention methods among all MSM, including those with HIV infection [41]. Beyond this, knowing the local epidemiology for particular STIs, including chlamydia, is helpful in understanding risk profiles for individual patients within broader sexual networks. Eliciting a comprehensive sexual history includes inquiring about number and sex of partners, HIV status of partners, use of safer sex methods (condoms, female condoms, dental dams, etc.), types of sexual activity (oral sex, anal sex, etc.), role in sexual partnerships (insertive vs. receptive), any associated drug use (including alcohol) and contexts of sexual encounters (bath houses, internet, etc.). Clinicians should routinely ask about common STI-associated symptoms including urethral discharge, dysuria, anal pain or discharge, genital or anal ulcers, swollen or painful lymph nodes, fevers, sweats and rash.

To reduce the risk of acquisition and transmission of HIV, the CDC specifies screening for STI that includes annual urethral/urine screening for both gonorrhea and chlamydia among sexually active MSM, pharyngeal gonorrhea cultures for MSM with oral-genital exposure, and rectal chlamydia and gonorrhea cultures for MSM who engage in receptive anal sex [41]. Despite the CDC's intentions and public health efforts to adhere to these guidelines, historically few STD clinics and gay men's health centers have offered rectal chlamydial screening for asymptomatic MSM [42]. One study that evaluated the prevalence of chlamydial and gonorrhea infections among MSM in San Francisco, Calif. [7], applied previously validated NAATs to specimens obtained from the pharynx, rectum and urethra. These investigators found that 85% of rectal gonorrhea and chlamydia occurred in asymptomatic men. Moreover, 53% of chlamydial infections occurred at nonurethral sites and would have been missed if only urethral/urine screening was performed. Finally, more than 70% of chlamydial infections would have been missed and left untreated if only gonorrhea testing occurred. Given that both gonorrhea and chlamydia increase the risk of HIV acquisition and transmission, settings that conduct STI testing should optimize screening and treatment of asymptomatic MSM at all relevant anatomic sites, ideally with the use of NAATs.

An expert consultation was held in January 2009 to review optimal laboratory diagnostic testing for chlamydia and gonorrhea. Of notable relevance for care related to MSM was a recommendation for clinicians and laboratories to utilize NAATs for detection of rectal and oropharyngeal infections. While these specimen types have not yet been cleared by the US Food and Drug Administration (FDA) for performance of NAATs, laboratories can achieve Clinical Laboratory Improvement Amendments compliance to satisfy regulations for testing (available at: http://www.aphl.org/aphlprograms/infectious/std/Documents/CTGCLabGuidelinesMeetingReport.pdf). One study designed to detect rectal and pharyngeal gonorrhea and chlamydia among MSM conducted targeted outreach in six gay community-based organizations in 2007 in five urban centers across the USA [43]. Out of 30,000 collected rectal and pharyngeal samples, 1,600 tested positive for gonorrhea or chlamydia. In Los Angeles, tests utilizing nucleic acid amplification detected 248 positive rectal specimens out of 1,841 tested (13.5% positive), affirming the high sensitivity of this testing and remarkable prevalence of this infection among MSM. Implementing NAAT testing at these sites for the purpose of screening MSM was viewed as highly feasible. Notably, although the pharynx is likely an important reservoir for gonorrhea, the role for chlamydia testing at this site is unclear and currently not recommended [44].

Lymphogranuloma Venereum

The L1, L2 and L3 serovars of *C. trachomatis* cause the disease known as lymphogranuloma venereum (LGV). These serovars differ from those (D through K) that cause the more common sexually transmitted chlamydial infections (urethritis and cervicitis). LGV has been steadily gaining clinical and public health attention over the past several years. In 2004, public health officials in the Netherlands reported a case of a young man with ulcerative proctitis caused by a 'rare strain' of *C. trachomatis* [45, 46]. There have been additional reports since that time, and, as of February 2006, the CDC had identified 27 cases of LGV as a cause for this condition. The current exact number of cases of LGV in the USA is unknown, owing largely to the challenges in its diagnosis (discussed further in this section). Historically, LGV has been recognized as an STI among travelers returning from the Caribbean or other tropical areas, but those cases generally run a benign course with finding of a mild genital ulcer followed by development of inguinal lymphadenopathy (buboes).

The majority of cases identified in the LGV outbreak described in 2004 occurred in HIV-infected MSM who reported unprotected anal sex. Many of these infections were not diagnosed until the condition had been well established. Because the clinical course of LGV proctitis can vary from indolent to severe, manifesting with bloody and purulent rectal discharge and tenesmus, the condition might not be suspected early during the course of illness and diagnosis can be delayed. Because the rectal symptoms of LGV can be quite severe, including perirectal abscesses, referral to a gastroenterologist for colonoscopy or sigmoidoscopy to rule out inflammatory bowel disease has sometimes preceded identification of the correct diagnosis.

Definitive diagnosis of LGV proctitis is challenging. While direct testing on rectal mucosal specimens for *C. trachomatis* is indicated, the FDA has approved only cell culture for this purpose. However, cell culture is not widely available, is expensive and is technically difficult to interpret. As stated earlier, NAAT is not FDA approved for rectal specimens, but may be used in laboratories that meet validation specifications. Information about the process to obtain this validation can be found at www.cdc.gov/std/. *C. trachomatis* serology (complement fixation titers >1:64) can support the diagnosis of LGV in an appropriate clinical context but is performed infrequently, is not standardized and requires a high level of expertise to interpret. It may also not perform as well in diagnosing rectal infections in men as it does upper genital tract infection in women.

Current clinical guidance from the CDC for clinicians, particularly those who care for HIV-infected MSM, emphasizes the need to be alert for rectal signs and symptoms suggestive of proctitis. Clinicians who suspect a case of LGV proctitis should seek expert advice from local public health authorities and infectious disease specialists on how to diagnose the condition effectively. Often, given lack of available local expertise, this is not possible. In these cases, an empiric course of therapy is warranted. LGV responds well to doxycycline, but the drug must be given for 3 weeks (100 mg orally twice daily), a longer course than that required for non-LGV chlamydial infection, to be effective.

Conclusion

The current literature indicates that women who report sex with women are at risk for genital chlamydial infection, and should benefit from screening and surveillance programs aimed at this common infection. Further investigation focusing on the frequency and types of sexual risk behaviors, provision of appropriate STI diagnostic testing and prevention counseling, labeling of sexual identity and sexual networks in this group is needed. Men who report sex with men continue to be a group at high risk for genitourinary and rectal chlamydial infection. Providers are responsible for taking comprehensive sexual histories, conducting thorough physical exams and testing both urethral and rectal sites for chlamydia. Finally, given the evolving and dynamic nature of sexual networks locally and globally, providers ought to be keenly aware of risks of LGV acquisition, have a low threshold to report suspicious cases to public health and empirically initiate therapy in the appropriate clinical settings.

References

1 Chandra A, Mosher WD, Copen C, Sionean C: Sexual behavior, sexual attraction, and sexual identity in the United States: data from the 2006–2008 National Survey of Family Growth. Natl Health Stat Report 2011;3:1–36.

2 Diamant AL, et al: Lesbians' sexual history with men: implications for taking a sexual history. Arch Intern Med 1999;159:2730–2736.

3 Lindley LL, et al: STDs among sexually active female college students: does sexual orientation make a difference? Perspect Sex Reprod Health 2008;40:212–217.

4 Goodenow C, et al: Dimensions of sexual orientation and HIV-related risk among adolescent females: evidence from a statewide survey. Am J Public Health 2008;98:1051–1058.

5 Koh A, et al: Sexual risk factors among self-identified lesbians, bisexual women, and heterosexual women accessing primary care settings. Sex Transm Dis 2005;32:563–569.

6 Mayer KH, Klausner JD, Handsfield HH: Intersecting epidemics and educable moments: sexually transmitted disease risk assessment and screening in men who have sex with men. Sex Transm Dis 2001; 28:464–467.

7 Kent CK, et al: Prevalence of rectal, urethral, and pharyngeal chlamydia and gonorrhea detected in 2 clinical settings among men who have sex with men: San Francisco, California, 2003. Clin Infect Dis 2005; 41:67–74.

8 Dean L, et al: Lesbian, gay, bisexual, and transgender health: findings and concerns. J Gay Lesbian Med Assoc 2000;4:102–151.

9 O'Hanlan KA, Crum CP: Human papillomavirus-associated cervical intraepithelial neoplasia following lesbian sex. Obstet Gynecol 1996;88(4 Pt 2):702–703.

10 Kellock D, O'Mahony CP: Sexually acquired metronidazole-resistant trichomoniasis in a lesbian couple. Genitourin Med 1996;72:60–61.

11 Marrazzo JM, Stine K, Koutsky LA: Genital human papillomavirus infection in women who have sex with women: a review. Am J Obstet Gynecol 2000; 183:770–774.

12 Tao G: Sexual orientation and related viral sexually transmitted disease rates among US women aged 15 to 44 years. Am J Public Health 2008;98:1007–1009.

13 Marrazzo JM, Stine K, Wald A: Prevalence and risk factors for infection with herpes simplex virus type-1 and -2 among lesbians. Sex Transm Dis 2003;30: 890–895.

14 Marrazzo JM, et al: Papanicolaou test screening and prevalence of genital human papillomavirus among women who have sex with women. Am J Public Health 2001;91:947–952.

15 Kwakwa HA, Ghobrial MW: Female-to-female transmission of human immunodeficiency virus. Clin Infect Dis 2003;36:e40–e41.

16 Marrazzo JM, et al: Characterization of vaginal flora and bacterial vaginosis in women who have sex with women. J Infect Dis 2002;185:1307–1313.

17 Singh D, Fine D, Marrazzo JM: *Chlamydia trachomatis* infection among women reporting sex with women screened in family planning clinics in the Pacific Northwest, 1997–2005. Am J Public Health 2011;101:1284–1290.

18 Gorgos L, Fine D, Marrazzo J: Chlamydia positivity in American Indian/Alaska Native women screened in family planning clinics, 1997–2004. Sex Transm Dis 2008;35:753–757.

19 Bailey JV, et al: Sexually transmitted infections in women who have sex with women. Sex Transm Infect 2004;80:244–246.

20 Marrazzo JM, Koutsky LA, Handsfield HH: Characteristics of female sexually transmitted disease clinic clients who report same-sex behaviour. Int J STD AIDS 2001;12:41–46.

21 Cochran SD, et al: Cancer-related risk indicators and preventive screening behaviors among lesbians and bisexual women. Am J Public Health 2001;91:591–597.

22 Mercer CH, et al: Women who report having sex with women: British national probability data on prevalence, sexual behaviors, and health outcomes. Am J Public Health 2007;97:1126–1133.

23 Einhorn L, Polgar M: HIV-risk behavior among lesbians and bisexual women. AIDS Educ Prev 1994;6: 514–523.

24 Marrazzo JM, Coffey P, Bingham A: Sexual practices, risk perception and knowledge of sexually transmitted disease risk among lesbian and bisexual women. Perspect Sex Reprod Health 2005;37:6–12.

25 Kurth AE, et al: A comparison between audio computer-assisted self-interviews and clinician interviews for obtaining the sexual history. Sex Transm Dis 2004;31:719–726.

26 Lemp GF, et al: Seroprevalence of HIV and risk behaviors among young homosexual and bisexual men. The San Francisco/Berkeley Young Men's Survey. JAMA 1994;272:449–454.

27 Marrazzo J, Cassells S, Ringwood K: Characteristics of young bisexual women's relationships with their male partners. 2006 National STD Prevention Conference, Jacksonville, Centers for Disease Control and Prevention, 2006.

28 Friedman SR, et al: Sociometric risk networks and risk for HIV infection. Am J Public Health 1997;87: 1289–1296.

29 Fethers K, et al: Sexually transmitted infections and risk behaviours in women who have sex with women. Sex Transm Infect 2000;76:345–349.

30 Saewyc EM, et al: Sexual intercourse, abuse and pregnancy among adolescent women: does sexual orientation make a difference? Fam Plann Perspect 1999; 31:127–131.

31 Bevier P, et al: Women at a sexually transmitted disease clinic who reported same-sex contact: their HIV seroprevalence and risk behaviors. Am J Public Health 1995;10:1366–1371.

32 Ness RB, et al: Bacterial vaginosis (BV) and the risk of incident gonococcal or chlamydial genital infection in a predominantly black population. Sex Transm Dis 2005;32:413–417.

33 Wiesenfeld HC, et al: Bacterial vaginosis is a strong predictor of *Neisseria gonorrhoeae* and *Chlamydia trachomatis* infection. Clin Infect Dis 2003;36:663–668.

34 Yoshimura K, et al: Can bacterial vaginosis help to find sexually transmitted diseases, especially chlamydial cervicitis? Int J STD AIDS 2009;20:108–111.

35 Fethers K: Is bacterial vaginosis a sexually transmitted infection? Sex Transm Infect 2001;77:390.

36 McCaffrey M, et al: Bacterial vaginosis in lesbians: evidence for lack of sexual transmission. Int J STD AIDS 1999;10:305–308.

37 Pinto VM, et al: Sexually transmitted disease/HIV risk behaviour among women who have sex with women. AIDS 2005;19(suppl 4):S64–S69.

38 Koumans EH, et al: The prevalence of bacterial vaginosis in the United States, 2001–2004; associations with symptoms, sexual behaviors, and reproductive health. Sex Transm Dis 2007;34:864–869.

39 Bailey JV, Farquhar C, Owen C: Bacterial vaginosis in lesbians and bisexual women. Sex Transm Dis 2004;31:691–694.

40 US Preventive Services Task Force: Screening for chlamydial infection: US Preventive Services Task Force recommendation statement. Ann Intern Med 2007;147:128–134.

41 Workowski KA, Berman S, Centers for Disease Control and Prevention: Sexually transmitted diseases treatment guidelines. MMWR Recomm Rep 2010; 59(RR-12):1–110.

42 Battle TJ, et al: Evaluation of laboratory testing methods for *Chlamydia trachomatis* infection in the era of nucleic acid amplification. J Clin Microbiol 2001;39:2924–2927.

43 Centers for Disease Control and Prevention: Clinic-based testing for rectal and pharyngeal *Neisseria gonorrhoeae* and *Chlamydia trachomatis* infections by community-based organizations – five cities, United States, 2007. MMWR Morb Mortal Wkly Rep 2009; 58:716–719.

44 Bernstein KT, et al: *Chlamydia trachomatis* and *Neisseria gonorrhoeae* transmission from the oropharynx to the urethra among men who have sex with men. Clin Infect Dis 2009;49:1793–1797.

45 Nieuwenhuis RF, et al: Resurgence of lymphogranuloma venereum in Western Europe: an outbreak of *Chlamydia trachomatis* serovar l2 proctitis in the Netherlands among men who have sex with men. Clin Infect Dis 2004;39:996–1003.

46 Nieuwenhuis RF, et al: Unusual presentation of early lymphogranuloma venereum in an HIV-1 infected patient: effective treatment with 1 g azithromycin. Sex Transm Infect 2003;79:453–455.

Devika Singh, MD, MPH
Harborview Medical Center
Box 359927, 325 Ninth Avenue
Seattle, WA 98104 (USA)
E-Mail dsingh@uw.edu

Black CM (ed): Chlamydial Infection: A Clinical and Public Health Perspective.
Issues Infect Dis. Basel, Karger, 2013, vol 7, pp 151–157 (DOI: 10.1159/000348767)

Lymphogranuloma Venereum: A Concise Outline of an Emerging Infection among Men Who Have Sex with Men

Henry J.C. de Vries[a, b, d] · Servaas Morré[c]

[a]Department of Dermatology, Academic Medical Centre, University of Amsterdam, [b]STI Outpatient Clinic,
Infectious Disease Cluster, Public Health Service Amsterdam, and [c]Department of Pathology, Laboratory
of Immunogenetics, VU University Medical Centre, Amsterdam, and [d]Centre for Infectious Disease Control,
National Institute of Public Health and the Environment, Bilthoven, The Netherlands

Abstract

Historically, lymphogranuloma venereum (LGV) was seen only in tropical areas as a sexually transmissible infection. In the last decades of the previous century, LGV was seen in countries with a moderate climate solely as an 'imported' disease. This changed in 2003, when the first cases of endemically acquired LGV proctitis were reported in the Netherlands among men who have sex with men (MSM), who were predominantly HIV positive. A disturbing association in this current epidemic is the high prevalence of hepatitis C among patients diagnosed with LGV. Since then, an ongoing epidemic in Western society has been revealed which has been dated back to 1981. In this chapter, diagnostics, treatment and common complications concerning LGV are discussed. Moreover, we focus on the epidemiological background of the recent epidemic of LGV among MSM in Western society and the associated risk factors. Early diagnosis is important to prevent irreversible late complications like anal strictures, mega colon and chronic fistulas. There is an urgent need for less expensive diagnostic assays for screening purposes to prevent more expansive transmission within the community. The microbial and immunological background of LGV infection in relation to HIV should be studied in detail and could help to explain the considerable number of asymptomatic LGV cases.

Epidemiology

Lymphogranuloma venereum (LGV) is caused by *Chlamydia trachomatis* biovars L1, L2 and L3, of which L2 is the most common serotype [1]. LGV is endemic in large parts of Africa, South-East Asia, Latin America and the Caribbean [2]. Until 2003 sporadic cases were reported in Europe and North America. These cases were mainly among seafarers, military and travelers who became infected during visits to LGV-endemic regions and were considered imported. In 1995 the rarer L1 biovar was identified in an outbreak in Seattle among men who have sex with men (MSM) with LGV proctitis [3].

Since 2003 multiple cases of LGV proctitis among MSM have been reported, starting in the Netherlands, followed by neighboring countries, other Western European countries and most recently in North America and Australia [4–6]. A molecular genetic retrospective study based on variation in the *ompA* gene showed that the LGV variant L2b (the Amsterdam variant) responsible for the epidemic in the Netherlands could be detected in rectal swabs from MSM who visited the city clinic in San Francisco back in 1981 [7, 8]. This finding proved that the LGV epidemic among MSM in the Western world was not a sudden outbreak but was a slow epidemic that had gone unnoticed for more than 20 years. Very recently we analyzed with multilocus sequence typing other regions of the *C. trachomatis* genome of LGV *C. trachomatis* strains from MSM in Europe and the USA [9]. The specimens from the 2003 outbreak in Europe were monoclonal. In contrast, several unique strains were detected in the USA dating back to the 1980s, including the variant circulating in Europe. This finding suggests a single source of origin for the LGV outbreak among MSM in Europe, possibly imported recently from the USA.

The current LGV epidemic due to L2b is confined to MSM of which the majority are coinfected with HIV (approximately 80%) and often other sexually transmitted infections, and also hepatitis C, which was up until recently not considered a sexually transmissible pathogen [10]. Because LGV is an ulcerative disease, the transmission of blood-borne diseases like hepatitis C, and also HIV, is possibly facilitated. Following the first reports in 2003 the epidemic is ongoing to date. On a weekly basis new cases of LGV are diagnosed at the outpatient clinic of the Health Service in Amsterdam [11]. The number of LGV cases among MSM is still increasing [12, 13]. Recent reports of endemically acquired LGV among heterosexual patients in France and the Netherlands could herald transmission outside the initial core groups and needs close monitoring [14, 15].

Clinical Presentation

LGV can cause several clinical syndromes of which the 'classical' inguinal syndrome and the anorectal syndrome are the most prevalent [16]. A third rare presentation is the pharyngeal syndrome affecting the mouth and throat [1]. The inguinal syndrome is characterized by genital ulcers. These are usually small, inconspicuous and short lived (they tend to heal within 1 week). Subsequently, inguinal lymphadenopathy can arise with the formation of buboes (fig. 1). If left untreated, inguinal LGV can lead to chronic genital inflammatory processes with fistulas, local destruction of the lymphatic drainage system resulting in genital lymphedema (elephantiasis). The anorectal syndrome is characterized by severe proctitis symptoms like anal cramps (tenesmus), pain, bloody discharge and constipation due to edema of the mucosal lining

de Vries · Morré

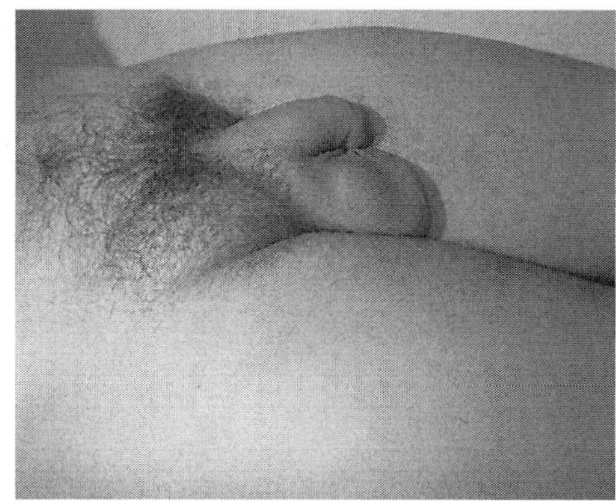

Fig. 1. Inguinal bubo formation, a sign of the inguinal LGV syndrome.

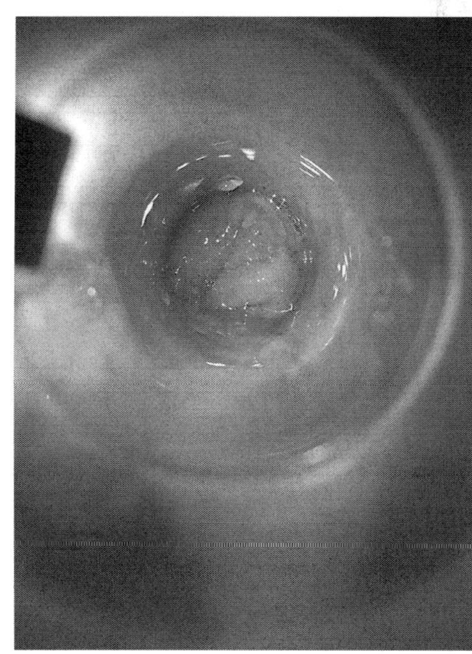

Fig. 2. Severe LGV proctitis upon anoscopic examination. Signs of edema, discharge and punctuate hemorrhagic lesions in the mucosal lining are present.

and underlying tissue (fig. 2). Also peri-anal painful ulceration can occur (fig. 3). Normally the anorectal syndrome is not accompanied by lymphadenopathy noticeable upon physical examination. However, with radiologic imagery techniques, lymphadenopathy in the pelvic area can be objectified.

Compared to proctitis caused by *C. trachomatis* trachoma biovars D-K, LGV proctitis is accompanied by much more severe complaints [1]. If left untreated, the anorectal syndrome can lead to anal strictures, which is a severe complication disabling the patient due to soiling, pain, constipation and the possible development of mega colon [17]. It has become apparent that LGV proctitis may closely resemble an

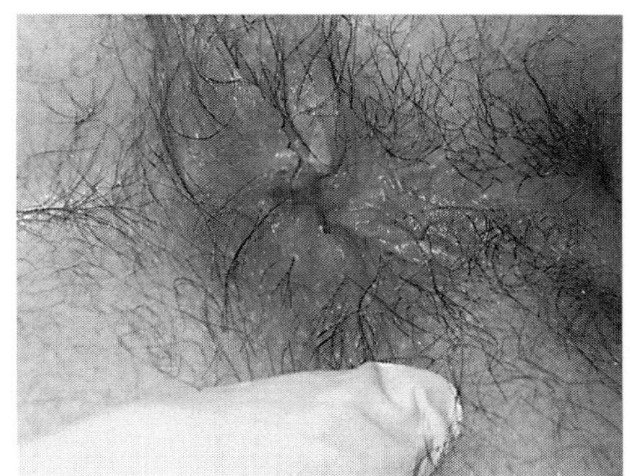

Fig. 3. Perianal ulcerations, as sometimes seen in MSM with anorectal LGV.

inflammatory bowel disease like Crohn's disease [18]. Delay of the correct diagnosis combined with initial clinical response to immunosuppressive therapy can lead to progression towards irreversible late complications. All LGV syndromes can be associated with systemic complaints like weight loss, arthritis and fever. In the present LGV epidemic among MSM, a considerable number of the patients with LGV proctitis are asymptomatic upon the time of diagnosis, possibly due to the HIV coinfection which accompanies most patients [7, 19]. Overall, the clinical manifestations of the L1 and the L2b strain seem less severe than those described in cases with the L2 biovar [3].

Diagnosis

The diagnosis of LGV is made on the detection of biovar-specific bacterial DNA in rectal specimens (in case anorectal LGV is suspected) or in genital ulcers or bubo aspirate (in case inguinal LGV is suspected). It is advised for budgetary reasons to follow a 2-step procedure. First, a commercially available pan *C. trachomatis* nucleic acid amplification test (NAAT) can be used to screen suspected samples [20]. Although all commercially available tests are not approved for extra-genital sites, a large body of literature supports the use of these tests for the detection of rectal chlamydia infections [4, 16, 19, 21]. Based on inhibitory factors it is advised to isolate pure nucleic acids out of the rectal samples instead of using sample preparation methods which only partially prepare samples for NAAT techniques. In case *C. trachomatis* is found, LGV biovar-specific DNA needs to be detected. For this purpose two 'in house' NAAT tests have been developed: a real-time PCR-based test that specifically detects all *C. trachomatis* LGV biovar strains by Morre et al. [22], and recently a real-time quadriplex PCR assay which incorporates an LGV-specific and a non-LGV-specific target sequence, a *C. trachomatis* plasmid target and the human RNase P gene as an internal control has been described by Chen et al. [23]. Both tests need real-time PCR equipment and are more laborious and expensive than most standard commercially available CT detection systems since they are regarded as typing assays. In case these requirements are not at hand a presumptive LGV diagnosis can be made using *Chlamydia*-specific serological assays [24]. An exeptionally high antibody titre in a patient with complaints supports LGV diagnosis. Nonetheless, a low titre does not rule out LGV, nor does a high titre in a patient without LGV symptoms prove LGV infection [7, 19]. Although it was stated that an elevated *Chlamydia*-specific IgA and IgG titre was associated with LGV [25], asymptomatic LGV infections require LGV-specific NAAT assays for proper diagnostics [26].

Treatment

The first choice of treatment for LGV is doxycycline 100 mg b.i.d. for 21 days [27]. We recently showed that a regimen of 21 days is required in LGV proctitis, since *C. trachomatis* RNA can persist up to 16 days under doxycycline therapy [28]. Erythromycin (500 mg q.i.d. for 21 days) is also effective but can cause more gastrointestinal side effects; it is second choice in case of pregnancy and if doxycycline is contraindicated. To date, there is insufficient data on the effectiveness of azithromycin for LGV and further controlled studies are required [29]. Cases of persisting and reactivated LGV after treatment with doxycycline standard therapy in HIV-positive patients have been reported [30, 31]. There is a need for antibiotic regimens with a shorter duration to improve patient therapy compliance. Contact tracing and contact treatment should be performed in all partners within the preceding 30 days before the complaints commenced.

Risk Factors in the Current Epidemic among MSM

The most important risk factors associated with LGV are HIV coinfection, unprotected anal sex with multiple partners and a history of multiple sexually transmitted infections [19]. Fisting (inserting a hand into the partner's anal canal) has also been suggested as a risk factor for emerging infections among MSM like LGV and hepatitis C virus [10]. Recently, a strong association of LGV proctitis and enema use before anal sex has been revealed by our group [32].

Conclusions

In the ongoing LGV epidemic among MSM in the Western world there is a need for better and cheaper screening tools to detect cases in larger groups of individuals at risk. This is of importance to prevent complications in the individual patient and to halt transmission in the community. Physicians should consider LGV in case MSM present with inguinal lymphadenopathy, genital ulceration or proctitis complaints. If chronic inflammatory bowel syndromes like Crohn's disease are considered, especially in MSM, LGV proctitis should always be excluded. Shorter antibiotic courses than the present ones of 21 days are needed to increase patient compliance to the treatment, but require large controlled clinical trials. Lastly, a deeper understanding of the microbial and immunological background of LGV infection in relation to HIV could shed light on the considerable number of asymptomatic LGV cases found.

Acknowledgements

The aims of this work are in line with the European EpiGenChlamydia Consortium which is supported by the European Commission within the Sixth Framework Programme through contract No. LSHG-CT-2007-037637. See www.EpiGenChlamydia.eu for more details about this consortium.

References

1 Perine PL, Stamm WE: Lymphogranuloma venereum; in Holmes KK, Sparling PF, Mardh PA, et al. (eds): Sexually Transmitted Diseases, ed 3. New York, McGraw-Hill, 1999, pp 423–432.

2 Herring A, Richens J: Lymphogranuloma venereum. Sex Transm Infect 2006;82(suppl 4):iv23–iv25.

3 Bauwens JE, Lampe MF, Suchland RJ, et al: Infection with *Chlamydia trachomatis* lymphogranuloma venereum serovar LI in homosexual men with proctitis: molecular analysis of an unusual case cluster. Clin Infect Dis 1995;20:576–581.

4 Halse TA, Musser KA, Limberger RJ: A multiplexed real-time PCR assay for rapid detection of *Chlamydia trachomatis* and identification of serovar L-2, the major cause of Lymphogranuloma venereum in New York. Mol Cell Probes 2006;20:290–297.

5 Nieuwenhuis RF, Ossewaarde JM, Gotz HM, et al: Resurgence of lymphogranuloma venereum in Western Europe: an outbreak of *Chlamydia trachomatis* serovar L2 proctitis in the Netherlands among men who have sex with men. Clin Infect Dis 2004;39: 996–1003.

6 Ward H, Martin I, Macdonald N, et al: Lymphogranuloma venereum in the United kingdom. Clin Infect Dis 2007;44:26–32.

7 Spaargaren J, Fennema HS, Morre SA, et al: New lymphogranuloma venereum *Chlamydia trachomatis* variant, Amsterdam. Emerg Infect Dis 2005; 11:1090–1092.

8 Spaargaren J, Schachter J, Moncada J, et al: Slow epidemic of lymphogranuloma venereum L2b strain. Emerg Infect Dis 2005;11:1787–1788.

9 Christerson L, de Vries HJ, de Barbeyrac B, et al: Typing of lymphogranuloma venereum *Chlamydia trachomatis* strains. Emerg Infect Dis 2010;16:1777–1779.

10 van de Laar TJ, Van der Bij AK, Prins M, et al: Increase in HCV incidence among men who have sex with men in Amsterdam most likely caused by sexual transmission. J Infect Dis 2007;196:230–238.

11 Koedijk FD, de Boer IM, de Vries HJ, et al: An ongoing outbreak of lymphogranuloma venereum in the Netherlands, 2006–2007. Euro Surveill 2007;12: E070419.

12 Ward H, Miller RF: Lymphogranuloma venereum: here to stay? Sex Transm Infect 2009;85:157.

13 de Vrieze NH, van Rooijen M, van der Loeff MF, de Vries HJ: Anorectal and inguinal lymphogranuloma venereum among men who have sex with men in Amsterdam, the Netherlands: trends over time, symptomatology and concurrent infections. Sex Transm Infect 2013, Feb 20 [Epub ahead of print].

14 Peuchant O, Baldit C, Le Roy C, et al: First case of Chlamydia trachomatis L2b proctitis in a woman. Clin Microbiol Infect 2011;17:E21–E23.

15 Verweij SP, Ouburg S, de Vries H, et al: The first case record of a female patient with bubonic lymphogranuloma venereum (LGV), serovariant L2b. Sex Transm Infect 2012;88:346–347.

16 Hamill M, Benn P, Carder C, et al: The clinical manifestations of anorectal infection with lymphogranuloma venereum (LGV) versus non-LGV strains of *Chlamydia trachomatis*: a case-control study in homosexual men. Int J STD AIDS 2007;18:472–475.

17 Pinsk I, Saloojee N, Friedlich M: Lymphogranuloma venereum as a cause of rectal stricture. Can J Surg 2007;50:E31–E32.

18 Soni S, Srirajaskanthan R, Lucas SB, et al: Lymphogranuloma venereum proctitis masquerading as inflammatory bowel disease in 12 homosexual men. Aliment Pharmacol Ther 2010;32:59–65.

19 Van der Bij AK, Spaargaren J, Morre SA, et al: Diagnostic and clinical implications of anorectal lymphogranuloma venereum in men who have sex with men: a retrospective case-control study. Clin Infect Dis 2006;42:186–194.

20 McMillan A, van Voorst Vader PC, de Vries HJ: The 2007 European Guideline (International Union against Sexually Transmitted Infections/World Health Organization) on the management of proctitis, proctocolitis and enteritis caused by sexually transmissible pathogens. Int J STD AIDS 2007;18:514–520.

21 Jalal H, Stephen H, Alexander S, et al: Development of real-time PCR assays for genotyping of *Chlamydia trachomatis*. J Clin Microbiol 2007;45:2649–2653.

22 Morre SA, Spaargaren J, Fennema JS, et al: Real-time polymerase chain reaction to diagnose lymphogranuloma venereum. Emerg Infect Dis 2005;11:1311–1312.

23 Chen CY, Chi KH, Alexander S, Ison CA, Ballard RC: A real-time quadriplex PCR assay for the diagnosis of rectal lymphogranuloma venereum (LGV) and non-LGV *Chlamydia trachomatis* infections. Sex Transm Infect 2008;84:273–276.

24 de Vries HJ, Smelov V, Ouburg S, et al: Anal lymphogranuloma venereum infection screening with IgA anti-*Chlamydia trachomatis*-specific major outer membrane protein serology. Sex Transm Dis 2010;37:789–795.

25 van der Snoek EM, Ossewaarde JM, van der Meijden WI, et al: The use of serological titres of IgA and IgG in (early) discrimination between rectal infection with non-lymphogranuloma venereum and lymphogranuloma venereum serovars of *Chlamydia trachomatis*. Sex Transm Infect 2007;83:330–334.

26 Smelov V, Morré SA, de Vries HJ: Are serological chlamydia-specific markers useful to detect asymptomatic cases of lymphogranuloma venereum proctitis? Sex Transm Infect 2008;84:77–78.

27 de Vries HJ, Morré SA, White JA, et al: European guideline for the management of lymphogranuloma venereum, 2010. Int J STD AIDS 2010;21:533–536.

28 de Vries HJ, Smelov V, Middelburg JG, et al: Delayed microbial cure of lymphogranuloma venereum proctitis with doxycycline treatment. Clin Infect Dis 2009;48:e53–e56.

29 McLean CA, Stoner BP, Workowski KA: Treatment of lymphogranuloma venereum. Clin Infect Dis 2007;44(suppl 3):S147–S152.

30 Richardson D, Goldmeier D: Lymphogranuloma venereum: an emerging cause of proctitis in men who have sex with men. Int J STD AIDS 2007;18:11–14.

31 Mechai F, de Barbeyrac B, Aoun O, et al: Doxycycline failure in lymphogranuloma venereum. Sex Transm Infect 2010;86:278–279.

32 de Vries HJ, Van der Bij AK, Fennema JS, et al: Lymphogranuloma venereum proctitis in men who have sex with men is associated with anal enema use and high-risk behavior. Sex Transm Dis 2008;35:203–208.

Henry J.C. de Vries
Department of Dermatology, Academic Medical Centre
PO Box 22700
NL–1100 DE, Amsterdam (The Netherlands)
E-Mail h.j.devries@amc.nl

Author Index